# DERMATOLOGY POSTGRADUATE MCQs AND REVISION NOTES

# DERMATOLOGY POSTGRADUATE MCQs AND REVISION NOTES

## James Halpern
### MRCP
*Specialty Registrar in Dermatology*
*University Hospital Birmingham*

Edited by
## Asad Salim
### FRCP
*Consultant Dermatologist*
*Countess of Chester NHS Trust*

Foreword by
## Celia Moss
*Professor of Paediatric Dermatology*
*Birmingham Children's Hospital*

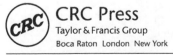

**CRC Press**
Taylor & Francis Group
Boca Raton  London  New York

CRC Press is an imprint of the
Taylor & Francis Group, an **informa** business

**Radcliffe Publishing Ltd**
18 Marcham Road
Abingdon
Oxon OX14 1AA
United Kingdom

www.radcliffe-oxford.com
Electronic catalogue and worldwide online ordering facility.

British Library Cataloguing in Publication Data

A catalogue record for this book is available from the British Library.

ISBN-13: 978 184619 440 5

The paper used for the text pages of this book is FSC certified. FSC (The Forest Stewardship Council) is an international network to promote responsible management of the world's forests.

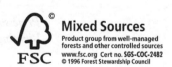

**Mixed Sources**
Product group from well-managed forests and other controlled sources
www.fsc.org Cert no. SGS-COC-2482
© 1996 Forest Stewardship Council

Typeset by Phoenix Photosetting, Chatham, Kent

# Contents

# Contents

# Foreword

There is a lot to learn in Dermatology. Trainees must master an enormous range of diagnoses in patients of all ages, a variety of clinical skills and laboratory investigations, and a great number of medical, physical and surgical treatments.

Earlier generations enjoyed a leisurely training, free to develop our own interests, dabbling here, exploring there, hopefully absorbing the essentials along the way. The idea of an exit exam was anathema, cramping inquisitive minds. The result was small pockets of erudition and large areas of woeful ignorance.

Over the last two decades, higher specialist training in dermatology has been compressed to four years. Targets and assessments became essential.

The Specialty Specific Examination (SCE) in dermatology, introduced in 2009, is only one of many hurdles UK dermatology trainees must jump before applying for a Certificate of Completion of Training in Dermatology. But compared to workplace-based assessments, this annual, centralised examination, run jointly by the British Association of Dermatologists and the Royal College of Physicians, seems the most daunting.

James Halpern has created this revision guide to demystify the SCE and to help dermatology trainees prepare for it. It is not a crammer. Browsing through it will help you understand the standards expected. Working through the examples will focus the mind and expose your weak spots. But remember that the exam is a means to an end, not an end in itself.

Celia Moss DM, FRCP, MRCPCH
Professor of Paediatric Dermatology
Birmingham Children's Hospital
*April 2010*

# Preface

Early in 2009 I embarked on revision for the Royal College of Physicians postgraduate specialist certificate examination in dermatology. Whilst revising I was frustrated by the lack of an appropriate revision aid. The great tomes of dermatology were simply too voluminous for exam revision and were not sufficiently up to date with the latest guidelines and treatments. Whereas undergraduate and introductory texts lacked the detail and depth required for a postgraduate examination. Many months ensued whilst I combined guidelines, read review articles and summarised chapters to produce my revision notes. It is these revision notes that form the basis of this book.

This book is not a textbook and should not be used as such; it is a revision aid for postgraduate examinations. Common and introductory topics are only briefly discussed and an understanding of basic dermatology is assumed. A 'best of five' multiple choice format has been used as this is now the mainstay of postgraduate examinations worldwide. Each chapter should be worked through in sequence as each question builds on the previous one to give the reader an encompassed understanding of the topic. Unlike similar books for other specialties this is not a 'cheat sheet' of questions taken from examinations, in fact an effort has been made to avoid duplication of exam questions. But candidates can be reassured that the detail in this book will answer the vast majority of exam questions.

It is my hope that reading this book will save postgraduates from making their own notes and allow them more time to concentrate on what is truly important – looking after patients.

**James Halpern**
*April 2010*

I am keen to continually improve this book and I would appreciate feedback from its readers. Please contact me at james_halpern@hotmail.com.

# About the authors

**James Halpern** is a third year dermatology registrar in the West Midlands deanery. He qualified from Birmingham medical school in 2003 having undertaken an intercalated degree in cell and molecular biology. Once qualified, he undertook training in general medicine at City Hospital Birmingham passing the MRCP in 2006. He joined the West Midlands dermatology rotation in 2007 and passed the specialist certificate examination in dermatology in 2009.

**Asad Salim** is a consultant dermatologist at Countess of Chester NHS Trust. He completed his dermatology training at West Midlands deanery in 2004. He has served on the West Midlands training committee for dermatology from 2005–08. His areas of interest in dermatology are paediatric dermatology, skin cancer, general dermatology and skin surgery.

# Acknowledgements

I would like to start by thanking those who nurtured and encouraged my interest in dermatology, if not for the kindness of these few people I would never have found my true vocation – Shireen Velangi, Camilo Diaz, Jai Bhat, Nigel Langford and all the staff of the dermatology department, City Hospital Birmingham. Special thanks must also go to all the consultants and registrars I have worked with at Stoke, Stafford, Selly Oak and Birmingham Children's Hospital.

In writing and editing this book I have received help from both colleagues and family. Without their help and support this book simply would not have been possible. I would like to thank Celia Moss for her support and encouragement, Ian Halpern for proof reading the manuscript and Clare Defty who has advised on content and question difficulty.

Last, but certainly not least, thanks must also go to my wife who has managed to juggle our young baby, spend untold time correcting my frankly atrocious spelling and grammar and advise on paediatric content.

# Chapter 1

# Eczematous and papulosquamous disorders

## QUESTIONS

**1** A six-month-old child presents with a symmetrical eczematous eruption on the cheeks, elbows and anterior aspects of the knees. The rash responds to a mild topical steroid cream but flares whenever the cream is stopped. What is the most likely cause of the rash:

A   seborrhoeic dermatitis
B   contact dermatitis to steroid cream
C   atopic eczema
D   food intolerance
E   acrodermatitis enteropathica.

**2** An eight-year-old boy of Indian descent presents to your clinic with ill-defined hypopigmented patches on his cheeks. He has a history of moderate atopic eczema controlled with 1% hydrocortisone ointment and a simple emollient. What is the most likely diagnosis:

A   melasma
B   pityriasis alba
C   steroid induced hypopigmentation
D   vitiligo
E   lepromatous leprosy.

**3** A 26-year-old man with a recent diagnosis of HIV infection presents with a rash and dandruff. The rash consists of small, scaly red patches and is prominent on the ears, face and trunk. What organism is most likely to have precipitated the rash:

A malassezia furfur
B streptococcus
C tinea mentagrophytes
D trichophyton rubrum
E tinea versicolor.

**4** You are asked to see an 88-year-old lady who has recently become resident in a nursing home. She gives a worsening history of a moderately itchy rash on her lower legs. On examination she has an eczematous rash with extreme xerosis and 'riverbed' cracking over the shins. Despite advice on using copious amounts of greasy emollients the rash does not improve. Which of these tests is likely to be the most useful for this lady:

A patch testing to emollients
B a full blood count with a blood film examination
C a skin biopsy
D skin scrapings for mycology
E thyroid function tests.

**5** A 55-year-old man presents with a new onset very itchy rash. On examination he has slightly weepy, eczematous, well defined annular patches worse on the limbs in an extensor distribution. He has had little benefit from regular clobetasone butyrate (Eumovate). Which treatment is the most appropriate:

A refined coal tar +/– dithranol
B 1% hydrocortisone ointment + aqueous cream
C oral prednisolone 40 mg/day for 5 days
D betamethasone/clioquinol (Betnovate-C) + antiseptic emollient
E PUVA phototherapy.

**6** An 82-year-old lady has been under your care for some time with a rash on her legs. She presented with a bilateral itchy, red, eczematous rash associated with haemosiderin deposition and varicosities. The rash was controlled with a combination of regular emollients, support stockings and betamethasone/neomycin ointment (Betnovate-N). Two years later she presents to you with a widespread eczematous eruption covering much of her body. What is most likely to have happened:

A   disseminated eczema with allergic contact dermatitis to neomycin
B   disseminated eczema with allergic contact dermatitis to betamethasone
C   secondary asteatotic eczema
D   superimposed zoster infection with koebnerization
E   development of nummular eczema.

**7** You review an eight-year-old boy with known behavioural problems and asthma who presents in shabby sportswear. His mum gives a six month history of worsening rash on the soles of his feet. The rash has not responded to a number of topical steroid preparations prescribed by his general practitioner. On examination over the balls and toepads of the feet the skin is dry, scaly and fissured with a glazed appearance. What treatment is most appropriate:

A   regular emollients only
B   a super-potent topical steroid
C   wear shoes less and use leather shoes rather than trainers
D   a short course of oral terbinafine
E   topical miconazole.

**8** A 52-year-old Englishman is admitted to coronary care after suffering an anterior myocardial infarction. After thrombolysis with streptokinase the patient is started on aspirin, clopidogrel, metoprolol, ramipril and simvastatin. During his recovery you are asked to see the patient as he has developed a rash. On examination he has multiple small beefy red plaques with silvery scale most prominent on the extensor surfaces. The patient's identical twin brother has psoriasis. What is the most likely diagnosis:

A he has caught psoriasis from another patient on the ward
B latent psoriasis precipitated by beta-blocker
C psoriasiform drug reaction to aspirin
D latent psoriasis precipitated by ACE inhibitor
E latent psoriasis precipitated by streptokinase.

**9** A 12-year-old boy attends your clinic as an emergency. The previous week shortly after a sore throat and coryzal illness, he has developed a rash. On examination he has a widespread rash consisting of multiple, small, deep red papules and plaques with some overlying scale. What initial treatment is most appropriate:

A admission to hospital and treatment with a potent topical steroid
B start on 1 mg/kg/day oral prednisolone
C work up for ciclosporin
D topical dithranol
E a coal tar preparation/mild topical steroid and consideration of UVB phototherapy.

**10** You are called to the antenatal ward to see a pregnant lady who has become quite unwell. On examination she has extensive areas of confluent erythema and numerous pustules. Despite being pyrexial initial swabs from a pustule grow no organisms. What is the likely diagnosis:

A generalised pustular psoriasis
B staphylococcal scalded skin syndrome
C toxic epidermal necrolysis
D eczema herpeticum
E gestational pemphigoid.

**11** A recently married 24-year-old nurse presents to you with a flare of palmo-plantar pustular psoriasis. She has previously maintained reasonable control of her condition with super potent topical steroids and vitamin D analogues. What would be the next reasonable step in treatment:

A   methotrexate
B   infliximab
C   acitretin
D   hand and foot PUVA
E   hydroxycarbamide.

**12** A 26-year-old woman presents with a rash. She describes the rash as occurring in crops with lesions tending to self resolve within a few weeks. On examination she has multiple erythematous to purple crusty papules with some small ulcers, vesicles and pustules. In some areas where lesions have resolved varioliform scarring has been left behind. A biopsy is taken that shows an interface dermatitis with necrotic keratinocytes, T-cell clonality studies show a predominantly CD8+ monoclonal infiltrate. What is the most likely diagnosis:

A   pityriasis lichenoides et varioliformis acuta (PLEVA)
B   pityriasis lichenoides chronic (PLC)
C   mycosis fungoides
D   guttate psoriasis
E   small plaque parapsoriasis.

**13** A 62-year-old man presents with diffuse erythroderma of gradual onset. He is systemically well. On examination follicular hyperkeratosis is seen on an erythematous base and there are large orange-red patches with distinctive islands of sparing. The palms and soles show an orange-red waxy keratoderma and there is fine diffuse scale on the scalp. The nails show a yellow-brown thickened nail plate with subungual debris. Which of the following treatments would you not consider for this patient:

A   hydroxychloroquine
B   methotrexate
C   acitretin
D   isotretinoin
E   combination methotrexate and acitretin.

**14** A 15-year-old girl presents with a two week history of a rash. She describes a single lesion appearing on her back that gradually enlarged over a few days, then multiple lesions appeared over the trunk and upper arms. The lesions are oval shaped, skin coloured and have a slightly raised margin. They vary from 2–4 cm in size, have central fine scale and a collarette of scale at the free edge. The lesions are asymptomatic and the patient is not unduly distressed by the rash. What is the appropriate course of action:

A   book the patient for UVB phototherapy
B   start a course of erythromycin
C   reassure the patient and advise a little sun exposure
D   start a topical steroid
E   give a course of oral prednisolone.

**15** A 52-year-old man is seen in clinic as an urgent referral. He gives a 2-week history of a spreading rash that now covers his whole body. The patient feels generally unwell, lethargic and thirsty. When you examine him he is shivering and has difficulty standing. He is erythrodermic with over 95% of his skin showing a non-specific confluent erythema. He has no history of skin disease and there are no clues to aetiology of the erythroderma in the history. What should you do next:

A   give an immediate dose of intramuscular corticosteroid and see him for review in one week
B   organise for daily emollients and dressings on the day case unit
C   admit to intensive care for consideration of inotropic support
D   admit the patient to the dermatology ward for assessment and stabilisation
E   take an urgent skin biopsy and organise for review when the histology is available.

**16** You review a 60-year-old woman who has been admitted to the ward with erythroderma. Her medical condition has been stabilised and a skin biopsy has been performed. She has no previous history of skin conditions and there are no clues to the aetiology on examination.

Her medications include salbutamol, simvastatin and hormone replacement therapy. Her skin biopsy shows a superficial lichenoid infiltrate composed mostly of lymphocytes some of which are atypical. What is the likely aetiology:

A   eczema
B   drug reaction to simvastatin
C   cutaneous T-cell lymphoma
D   sofa dermatitis
E   eruptive lichenoid keratosis.

**17** A 32-year-old female pharmacist presents with hand dermatitis. On examination her hands are dry and cracked with erythema and mild paronychia. At work she wears vinyl gloves whenever handling medicines and washes her hands regularly. She has no particular hobbies as she is busy with her three young children. What is the likely diagnosis:

A   irritant hand dermatitis
B   atopic hand dermatitis
C   allergic contact dermatitis to vinyl gloves
D   allergic contact dermatitis to medications
E   pompholyx eczema.

**18** The emergency department rings you for advice about a patient who claims to have an allergy to corticosteroids. The patient has been admitted with an exacerbation of inflammatory bowel disease and the team are keen to start systemic steroids. You have the patient's recent patch testing results to hand which showed a 3+ reaction to tixocortol-21-pivalate, the patient is awaiting further patch testing to the steroid series. Which of the following steroids is likely to be the safest:

A   hydrocortisone
B   methylprednisolone
C   dexamethasone
D   prednisolone
E   diflucortolone.

**19** You are asked to see a 12-year-old girl in the emergency department. She has bizarre configurations of erythema, oedema and bullae on her exposed arms and legs. Three days previously she had been playing in a field on a hot summer's day. You suspect a diagnosis of phytophotodermatitis. Which of the following plants is the most likely culprit:

A   urticaceae (nettle family)
B   asteraceae (thistle family)
C   solanaceae (chilli pepper family)
D   apium graveolens (celery)
E   toxicodendron radicans (poison ivy).

**20** Whilst on holiday in Thailand an 18-year-old girl has a henna tattoo of a dragon drawn on her right forearm by a beach vendor. Three days later her tattoo becomes progressively more inflamed and sore to the point of developing bullae. When she sees you three months later the reaction and henna have faded but an area of postinflammatory pigmentation remains. What important information should you give the patient:

A   now the reaction has settled it is safe to get another henna tattoo
B   it will be safe to get another henna tattoo in six months
C   she needs to carry an adrenalin containing pen as she is at risk of anaphylaxis
D   she must not use permanent hair dyes in the future
E   she must avoid all henna containing products in the future.

# ANSWERS

## 1 C. Atopic eczema

This child is likely to have simple atopic eczema. The pattern of atopic eczema is dependent on the age of the patient with classical flexural eczema often not appearing until later. As with any inflammatory dermatoses when topical treatments are stopped the rash will flare up soon afterwards.

**Table 1.1** Typical distributions of atopic eczema according to age

| Type | Age | Areas of skin affected |
|---|---|---|
| Infantile | 2 months–5 years | Facial, scalp, extensor surface of limbs, nappy area often spared |
| Childhood | 2–12 years | Antecubital fossa, popliteal fossa, posterior neck, wrist and hands |
| Adult | 12 years+ | Flexural surfaces of limbs, may be extensive and favour head or hands |

The description of the rash is not typical of seborrhoeic dermatitis which presents in infants with greasy scale and a predilection for the face and scalp. Contact dermatitis to a steroid is unlikely in such a young age group and does not fit with the rash flaring when treatment is stopped. Acrodermatitis enteropathica is a rash related to zinc deficiency that presents as an eczematous eruption favouring the face and nappy area; in this case the nappy area is not involved. The role of food intolerance in atopic eczema is highly controversial; in this case there is no mention of specific foods exacerbating the rash and the rash is typical of simple atopic eczema.

## 2 B. Pityriasis alba

Pityriasis alba is an uncommon feature of atopic dermatitis that presents in children and adolescents. Ill-defined hypopigmented patches occur, often on the face in a symmetrical distribution frequently on the cheeks. It is more common in patients with atopy and darkly pigmented skin. The patches represent a significant cosmetic challenge but do tend to resolve over time. There is no effective treatment for this condition.

Melasma is a condition of hyperpigmentation, with dark patches appearing on the face of patients with pigmented skin. It is associated with pregnancy and the oral contraceptive pill. Vitiligo is amelanotic rather than hypopigmented, with no melanin occurring within the areas affected. Vitiligo is characterised by sharply demarcated borders unlike pityriasis alba. Steroid induced hypopigmentation may occur but it is unlikely in a child using a mild strength steroid preparation. Patients with lepromatous leprosy tend to present with many skin lesions that may be hypopigmented and have reduced sensation.

### 3 A. Malassezia furfur

This patient is presenting with seborrhoeic dermatitis with a typical distribution affecting the scalp, ears, face, chest and intertriginous areas. There is a strong association between HIV infection and severe, treatment resistant seborrhoeic dermatitis. The aetiology of seborrhoeic dermatitis is complicated with interplay between overactive sebaceous glands, abnormal sebum production and malassezia furfur. Malassezia furfur, previously known as pityrosporum ovale, is a commensal yeast which can be isolated from the skin lesions of seborrhoeic dermatitis. Treatment of the yeast with anti-mycotic agents improves the rash of seborrhoeic dermatitis as do mild topical steroids, emollients and tar based therapies.

Tinea mentagrophytes and trichophyton rubrum are the most common organisms responsible for superficial fungal infections of the skin such as tinea pedis. They have no particular association with seborrhoeic dermatitis. Tinea versicolor is another superficial skin infection by the yeast malassezia furfur. It presents with mildly scaly hypo and hyperpigmented patches on the skin of young adults. The typical skin infection by streptococcus is impetigo presenting with superficial, stuck-on, honey coloured crusts overlying erosions.

### 4 E. Thyroid function tests

This elderly patient is presenting with asteatotic eczema, also known as eczema craquelé. This form of eczema is most common in elderly patients and results from extreme xerosis. It mostly occurs on the shins, flanks and axillae as a dry, scaly rash with cracking giving the appearance of a dry riverbed. It is exacerbated by low humidity and excessive washing of dry, frail skin. The skin changes related to hypothyroidism also predispose to xerosis and subsequent asteatotic eczema.

Patch testing is not unreasonable in asteatotic eczema as sensitisation to medicaments does occur, but this is less likely when using greasy thick emollients. There is no association with haematological disorders and secondary fungal infection is rare. Although a skin biopsy may help by confirming the diagnosis, it is an invasive procedure complicated by poor healing in the legs of elderly patients.

## 5 D. Betamethasone/clioquinol (Betnovate-C) + antiseptic emollient

This patient gives a typical history and examination findings of discoid eczema, also known as nummular dermatitis. Discoid eczema presents with well demarcated annular eczematous patches measuring 1–3 cm diameter, occurring almost exclusively on the extremities. The lesions are very itchy and may either be acutely inflamed with vesicles and weeping, or chronic and lichenified. Discoid eczema is also called microbial eczema as secondary bacterial infection seems to play a significant role in the pathology of the disorder. Initial treatment is with potent topical steroids and topical antimicrobials.

Light therapy is extremely effective in the treatment of discoid eczema but this is usually a second line treatment and narrow band UVB is used in preference to Psoralen plus UVA (PUVA). Tar is also an effective treatment for discoid eczema but steroids tend to be used in preference as a first line therapy. Dithranol is not used to treat eczema. Short courses of oral steroids are not recommended as discoid eczema is a chronic condition and discontinuation of oral steroids often results in a severe flare of disease. Hydrocortisone is a mild topical steroid and is not strong enough to treat this condition. Aqueous cream is also a poor choice as it is an ineffective emollient and contains potential sensitising agents.

## 6 A. Disseminated eczema with allergic contact dermatitis to neomycin

This elderly lady initially presented with venous eczema, also known as statis dermatitis. This form of eczema presents as a red itchy rash developing in an area of longstanding venous hypertension. Often on the legs of elderly women the eczema is associated with haemosiderin deposition, varicosities, oedema, induration, atrophie blanche and lipodermatosclerosis. Treatment is both of the eczema itself with topical steroids and emollients and of the venous hypertension with compression therapy.

The patient has subsequently developed disseminated eczema, also known as an Id reaction or autosensitisation dermatitis. This is where widespread secondary lesions of eczema occur distant to the primary site. The commonest cause of disseminated eczema is an allergic contact dermatitis complicating stasis dermatitis. In this case the patient has developed an allergic contact dermatitis to neomycin which is a more common sensitiser than betamethasone. The pattern of the rash is not typical for asteatotic or discoid eczema and eczema does not koebnerize.

## 7 C. Wear shoes less and use leather shoes rather than trainers

This young boy is presenting with juvenile plantar dermatosis. The history is of an atopic patient with a chronic eczematous rash on his feet that has not responded to topical steroids. Juvenile plantar dermatosis affects atopic prepubertal children from the age of three years when they start to wear shoes most of the time. It is thought to arise due to the humid environment created within impermeable shoes made of plastic and rubber. Treatment is advice on wearing breathable socks and leather shoes and allowing the socks to dry whenever possible. Emollients and keratolytics may be used to complement this advice, topical steroids are not needed and there is no fungal component to this condition.

## 8 B. Latent psoriasis precipitated by beta-blocker

This gentleman has a rash consisting of beefy red plaques and overlying silvery scale, a classical description of chronic plaque psoriasis. Psoriasis affects 1–2% of the world's population with a higher prevalence in Western Europe and America and a lower prevalence in Africans, Chinese and Native Americans. The genetics of psoriasis are complicated and polygenic but are a significant risk factor for developing the disorder. A monozygotic twin such as this patient has a 73% chance of developing psoriasis if his twin has the condition.

Triggering events that can precipitate latent psoriasis:
- cutaneous injury – the Koebner phenomenon
- infections – particularly streptococci, HIV
- psychogenic stress
- endocrine factors – pregnancy, hypocalcaemia
- drugs – beta-blockers, lithium, anti-malarial drugs, interferon.

In this question the likely precipitants are the psychogenic stress of the myocardialinfarction and beta-blockers. Psoriasis is not infectious and cannot be caught. The other drugs postulated are not known precipitators of psoriasis.

## 9 E. A coal tar preparation/mild topical steroid and consideration of UVB phototherapy

This young patient is presenting with guttate psoriasis following a probable streptococcal sore throat. Guttate psoriasis is most common in children and often follows a streptococcal infection. In children the prognosis is excellent with most cases resolving in a few weeks to months. In adults the prognosis is more guarded with many cases becoming chronic. If antibiotics are given early to treat the infection this can also resolve the rash. If the rash has developed it often responds well to topical coal tar, mild topical steroids and light therapy.

Potent topical steroids and oral prednisolone risk precipitating an unstable pustular psoriasis and should be avoided. Dithranol should only be applied to psoriatic plaques, avoiding normal skin, it would be impossible to apply to guttate disease. Ciclosporin is extremely effective in treating psoriasis but has many side effects and should be reserved for resistant cases.

## 10 A. Generalised pustular psoriasis

The history is of an unwell, pyrexial patient with an extensive erythematous rash and multiple sterile pustules. This is a typical presentation of generalised pustular psoriasis, an unusual manifestation of psoriasis that may be triggered by pregnancy. Other triggers include rapid tapering of systemic corticosteroids, hypocalcaemia and infections. The rash is characterised by erythema and an epidermal neutrophilic infiltrate causing multiple sterile pustules. Patients can be quite unwell and pyrexial. There is an overlap between this condition and acute generalised exanthematous pustulosis (AGEP) a pustular drug eruption. Treatment options include retinoids, ciclosporin and light therapy.

Staphylococcal scalded skin syndrome more commonly presents in children with thin walled blisters rather than pustules. Toxic epidermal necrolysis is characterised by sheets of epidermal detachment and mucous membrane involvement. Eczema herpeticum occur on a background of eczema and has vesicles rather than pustules. Gestational pemphigoid presents with itchy urticated plaques that form thick-walled blisters.

## 11 D. Hand and foot PUVA

Palmo-plantar pustular psoriasis is characterised by multiple sterile pustules and yellow-brown macules on the palms and soles. Only a small minority of patients have psoriasis elsewhere on the skin. The condition is more common in smokers and can be worsened by stress and infections. It can be associated with sterile inflammatory bone lesions and neutrophilic dermatoses. Treatment consists of topical agents, often under occlusion, hand and foot PUVA and systemic agents.

In this case you would be concerned about the patient falling pregnant during treatment. As methotrexate, acitretin and hydroxycarbamide are all teratogenic they would only be used with extreme caution. Although early data seems to show that Infliximab may be safe in pregnancy most clinicians would consider it a second or third line agent. In this case hand and foot PUVA gives a good compromise between drug efficacy and potential adverse events.

## 12 A. Pityriasis lichenoides et varioliformis acuta (PLEVA)

Pityriasis lichenoides et varioliformis acuta (PLEVA) and pityriasis lichenoides chronic (PLC) are considered to be two ends of the same disease spectrum. Both are characterised by recurrent crops of self-resolving erythematous papules. The lesions of PLEVA are more acute and tend to be crusty, vesicular and pustular whereas PLC tends to be more chronic and scaly. In reality few patients are at one end of the spectrum and most show a mixture of features. T-cell clonality is seen in both disorders and they may be considered as T-cell lymphoproliferative disorders. Treatment consists of topical steroids, coal tar products, antibiotics and light therapy.

The recurrent crops of PLEVA/PLC are quite characteristic and exclude other conditions such as mycosis fungoides and guttate psoriasis. Parapsoriasis is a related T-cell lymphoproliferative disorder that is considered by some to be a precursor to mycosis fungoides. It presents with chronic, asymptomatic scaly patches.

## 13 A. Hydroxychloroquine

This patient is presenting with clinical features consistent with pityriasis rubra pilaris (PRP). Some of the characteristic features include follicular papules on an erythematous base, islands of sparing and orange palmar-plantar keratoderma. As in this case the disorder can develop into an erythroderma. There are five types of PRP of which the adult type is commonest, childhood and inherited forms also exist. The classical adult variant of PRP normally resolves in 3–5 years. Histologically alternating orthokeratosis and parakeratosis is seen. Although no large scale randomised control trials exist, patients are often treated with retinoids and/or methotrexate. Hydroxychloroquine is not a recognised treatment.

## 14 C. Reassure the patient and advise a little sun exposure

This young girl gives a typical history of a herald patch appearing on her back followed by the development of pityriasis rosea. Pityriasis rosea is a self limiting eruption that affects young adults. It is often asymptomatic or mildly pruritic. The rash favours the trunk and proximal extremities and usually resolves in 6–8 weeks. It is thought that the rash is precipitated by a viral infection, possibly of the herpes virus family. In dark skin the rash tends to be hyperpigmented and less common variants can be inverse, vesicular, purpuric or pustular.

In this case as the rash is asymptomatic it is best not treated although a small amount of sun exposure may hasten its resolution. If the rash was itchy then symptomatic relief may be obtained using a topical steroid cream and oral antihistamines. Erythromycin and UVB phototherapy have both been used in resistant cases. There is no indication for oral corticosteroids.

## 15 D. Admit the patient to the dermatology ward for assessment and stabilisation

This middle-aged patient is presenting with rapid onset erythroderma and systemic upset. He is shivering due to loss of thermoregulatory control and is dehydrated leading to postural hypotension and thirst. He may also be suffering from other complications of erythroderma including tachycardia, protein loss, peripheral oedema and secondary infection.

As the patient is systemically unwell he needs admission to hospital for assessment and stabilisation of his medical condition. He is not unwell enough to require support from the intensive care unit, although elderly patients and patients with other medical co-morbidities may become this unwell. Systemic corticosteroids are used in erythroderma caused by for example, a drug reaction, but at this early stage it is important to first exclude conditions such as erythrodermic psoriasis in which systemic corticosteroids may be contraindicated.

## 16 C. Cutaneous T-cell lymphoma

In this case the cause of the woman's erythroderma is not immediately apparent. She has no previous history of skin disease and the skin biopsy is not typical of eczema or psoriasis, the two commonest causes of erythroderma in adults.

Common causes of erythroderma in adults:
- psoriasis
- atopic dermatitis
- drug reactions
- idiopathic
- cutaneous T-cell lymphoma.

Common causes of erythroderma in children and neonates:
- atopic dermatitis
- seborrhoeic dermatitis
- psoriasis
- inherited ichthyoses
- immunodeficiency
- infection.

Given this scenario it is important to carefully examine the patient's drug history; in this case none of her medications are strongly associated with erythrodermic drug reactions.

Medications associated with erythrodermic drug reactions:
- allopurinol
- beta-lactam antibiotics
- anti-epileptic medications
- gold
- sulphonamides.

The most likely diagnosis is cutaneous T-cell lymphoma given the histology of a lichenoid interface dermatitis and the presence of atypical lymphocytes. A significant proportion of cases labelled 'idiopathic' subsequently develop cutaneous T-cell lymphoma, it is important to follow these patients up and consider repeat skin biopsies.

## 17 A. Irritant hand dermatitis

Hand dermatitis is difficult to assess and requires a meticulous history. In this case there are a number of clues pointing towards the diagnosis of irritant hand dermatitis. The patient works as a pharmacist and is regularly washing her hands. She also has young children and is likely to be doing a lot of 'wet work' at home. Lastly she has mild paronychia, a low grade inflammation/infection around the nails that is also associated with 'wet work'.

Allergic contact dermatitis remains a possibility and although given the history this is less likely, it would not be unreasonable to organise patch testing for this patient. Pompholyx is an endogenous eczema characterised by vesicles and bullae on the palms and soles associated with seasonal exacerbations.

## 18 C. Dexamethasone

Topical corticosteroid allergy is rare and usually presents as treatment failure or worsening of a rash when a steroid cream is applied. Very rarely this may also present as allergy to systemic steroids given orally or by injection. Tixocortol-21-pivalate is commonly used as a steroid marker of allergic contact dermatitis, this alone picks up over 90% of steroid reactions. A positive reaction often indicates allergy to class A steroids – hydrocortisone, prednisolone, diflucortolone, methylprednisolone and prednicarbate. Patients with suspected steroid allergy should be patch tested to a steroid series and individual steroid preparations to elicit which steroids are safe to use. Four classes of steroid are recognised with cross reactivity commonly occurring within particular groups.

**Table 1.2** Classes of corticosteroids

| Group | Corticosteroids |
| --- | --- |
| Group A | Hydrocortisone acetate, cortisone, methylprednisolone, prednisolone, tixocortol and diflucortolone |
| Group B | Triamcinolone, halcinonide, fluocinonide, desonide, budesonide, amcinonide |
| Group C | Betamethasone, dexamethasone, fluocortolone |
| Group D | Hydrocortisone butyrate, clobetasone, clobetasol, betamethasone valerate, fluocortolone, prednicarbate, alclometasone |

There are a small number of other agents which can cause a topical allergic contact dermatitis and a systemic response when taken orally. For example, allergy to topical neomycin can lead to a systemic response to oral streptomycin and allergy to topical sorbic acid can lead to a systemic response to some food preservatives.

## 19 D. Apium graveolens (celery)

There are a number of non-phytophoto dermatological reactions that may occur from contact with plants as shown in Table 1.3.

**Table 1.3** Non-phytophoto cutaneous reactions from plants

| Mechanism of action | Description |
|---|---|
| Allergic contact dermatitis | A true allergic contact dermatitis can occur to plants, most commonly members of the anacardiaceae family which includes poison ivy and poison oak |
| Toxin mediated contact urticaria | Plants with sharp hairs that implant chemicals such as histamine and serotonin causing an urticarial response, most commonly stinging nettles |
| Mechanical irritant dermatitis | Spines and thorns cause a penetrating injury, commonly prickly pears, thistles and cacti |
| Chemical irritant dermatitis | Chemical irritants derived from plants, commonly calcium oxalate found in daffodil bulbs, hyacinth and rhubarb. Capsaicin in hot peppers is another example |

Phytophotodermatitis occurs when a plant derived chemical, commonly psoralen, comes in contact with the skin and is activated by UVA light. This results in a phototoxic reaction consisting of erythema, blistering and delayed hyperpigmentation. The cutaneous features often start 24 hours after exposure and peak at 72 hours. Most cases of phytophotodermatitis are due to contact with two families of plants – apiaceae and rutaceae. The apiaceae family includes cow parsley, celery, fennel and parsnip. The rutaceae family includes citrus fruits such as lime and orange.

**20 D. She must not use permanent hair dyes in the future**
This history is suggestive of an allergic contact dermatitis to paraphenylenediamine (PPD) a component of temporary tattoos. The patient developed a reaction three days after the tattoo was applied which is suggestive of a type IV allergic reaction to a compound she was not previously sensitised to. In this case the reaction was severe with bullae and postinflammatory hyperpigmentation. Patch testing would be the investigation of choice to confirm the diagnosis of PPD allergy.

PPD is most commonly used in permanent hair dyes, it is also found in textile dyes, darkly coloured cosmetics and inks. Given the severity of the original reaction it is likely that the patient will have a severe type IV allergic reaction to permanent hair dyes and these should be avoided along with other PPD containing products. She is not allergic to henna itself and as long as the henna product does not contain PPD it should be safe to use. The risk of a type IV PPD reaction causing anaphylaxis is small and she does not need to carry an adrenalin containing pen.

**Table 1.4** Common positive reactions on patch testing and their relevance

| Allergen | Relevance |
| --- | --- |
| Nickel | The commonest positive on patch testing but up to 50% of reactions may be irritant rather than allergic.* Patients are often sensitised when their ears are pierced. Nickel is found in jewellery, belt buckles, jeans studs and as a coating for white gold |
| Gold | Often associated with other metal allergies. May have a relevance to gold based pharmaceuticals |
| Cobalt | Associated with other metal allergies especially nickel and chromium. It is found in other metals as an alloy, ceramics, cement, cosmetics, paints, resins and hair dyes. Occupational allergy is seen in bricklayers and potters |
| Potassium dichromate | Chromium itself in non-allergenic but its salts may cause allergy and are found in wet cement, chrome, tanned leather, welding fumes, cutting oils and paint |
| Fragrance mix | A mixture of fragrances that detects ~75% of fragrance allergies, if positive patients should avoid fragrances, scents and perfumes |
| Balsam of Peru | A naturally occurring fragrance that is used in a number of products. There is cross reactivity with some spices such as cloves and cinnamon |
| Neomycin | A common medicament, neomycin is used as a topical antibiotic in creams, eye drops and ear drops |
| Fusidic acid | A topical antibiotic that may induce allergy |
| Caine mix | Caine mix contains three anaesthetics used in topical preparations – benzocaine, dibucaine hydrochloride and tetracaine hydrochloride, allergy to topical anaesthetics are well recognised |
| Lanolin | Commonly used in emollients and cosmetics. Patients may develop allergy to the wool alcohol component of lanolin |
| Thimerosal | A preservative used in vaccines, contact lens solutions, ear and eye drops and antiseptics. A positive reaction often has little clinical relevance |

*continued*

**Table 1.4** *continued*

| | |
|---|---|
| Formaldehyde | Formaldehyde itself is rarely used these days but a positive test is relevant to formaldehyde releasing preservatives which are widely used in cosmetics, medications, textiles, paints and resins. 'Wrinkle resistant' clothes are a notable source of formaldehyde releasing resins. Quaternium 15 is another notable formaldehyde releasing agent used as a biocide in antiseptics |
| Other preservatives | Other preservatives are used in a number of products including cosmetics and can cause allergy. These include parabens mix, methyldibromoglutaronitrile phenoxyethanol, methylchloroisothiazolinone, methylisothiazolinone (Kathon CG) |
| Rubber based products | Allergy can occur to rubber, latex and rubber accelerators. Patients can be patch tested to thiuram mix, mercapto mix, carba mix, and mercaptobenzothiazole |
| Paraphenylenediamine (PPD) | *See* above |
| Steroids | *See* question 18 |
| Nail allergens | Patients may develop allergy to a number of compounds used in nail polish, artificial nails, nail glues and film formers. Examples which may be patch tested include the acrylates and tosylamide formaldehyde resin |
| Adhesives | A number of potential adhesive allergens can be tested including colophony, epoxy resins, formaldehyde resins and rosin |
| Plants | Allergy to plants can be elicited using sesquiterpene lactone mix, primin and dedicated plant series. *See* question 19 |

*In this table allergy refers to a type IV allergic contact dermatitis.

# Chapter 2

# General dermatology

## QUESTIONS

**21** A 20-year-old Indian patient presents with white patches of skin that have developed around his mouth and eyes. He has a past history of diabetes and you note that where a patch crosses the left eyebrow the hair is white. You suspect a diagnosis of vitiligo but also consider other causes of acquired hypopigmentation. Which of the following would not be in your differential diagnosis:

A  pinta
B  leprosy
C  piebaldism
D  pityriasis alba
E  post-inflammatory from lupus.

**22** A 37-year-old man presents with widespread rash including his palms and soles. On examination the rash consists of multiple annular lesions measuring 1–3 cm in diameter with a targetoid appearance, there is no mucosal involvement. The rash has been present for over six months occurring intermittently following crops of painful mouth ulcers. Which of the following treatment options would you recommend:

A  2 week course of tapering prednisolone
B  long term low dose aciclovir
C  6 week course of amoxicillin
D  admit for IV immunoglobulins
E  start ciclosporin.

**23** A 42-year-old woman presents to the emergency department with a rash. On examination she has a widespread erythematous eruption with haemorrhagic oral crusting and conjunctivitis. The next day on the ward she becomes very unwell with sheets of skin loss and a positive nikolsky sign. Which of her drugs is most likely to be responsible:

A   codeine phosphate
B   oral contraceptive pill
C   propranolol
D   ciclosporin
E   allopurinol.

**24** You review a 58-year-old woman who has been referred with an urticarial type rash. On review of her medications which of the following may be exacerbating the urticaria:

A   doxepin
B   aspirin
C   phenytoin
D   promethazine
E   methyldopa.

**25** A middle-aged man presents with a dry rash worse on his legs. On examination he has dry, thickened scaly skin consistent with ichthyosis. His skin problem has only been present for a few months and the patient is adamant that his skin was normal in childhood. Which of the following investigations would be most useful:

A   HIV test
B   genetic testing for keratin mutations
C   patch testing
D   24-hour urinary amino acid testing
E   direct immunofluorescence of a skin biopsy.

**26** A 55-year-old man presents with an itchy plaque on his calf. On examination there is a well demarcated plaque with scaling, excoriation and lichenification consistent with lichen simplex. Which of the following is another common site where lichen simplex is seen:

A knee
B plantar foot
C ear
D cheek
E wrist.

**27** A 14-year-old boy presents with sudden onset acne and systemic upset. On examination he has severe inflamed, ulcerated, nodular acne affecting his face, shoulders, chest and back. He is pyrexial, lethargic and describes painful joints. Which of the following features would you not expect to find in this patient:

A sterile meningitis
B osteolytic bone lesions of the clavicle
C hepatomegaly
D arthralgia
E erythema nodosum.

**28** A middle-aged patient presents with a monomorphic acneiform eruption covering much of his back. He had mild acne as a teenager but has had good skin since. Which of his medications is most likely to be responsible for the rash:

A paroxetine
B methotrexate
C lithium
D simvastatin
E omeprazole.

**29** An elderly man presents with a rash on his face and changes to his nose. On examination he has papules, pustules and rhinophyma typical of rosacea. In what ethnic group is rosacea most common:

A Southern European
B Northern European
C South-East Asian
D Afro-Caribbean
E South Asian.

**30** A 34-year-old woman presents with an itchy rash on her wrists and ankles. On examination there is a purple rash consisting of polygonal papules and overlying white lacy streaks. Further examination reveals a white lacy eruption on the buccal and vulval mucosa. What would be your first line treatment for this patient:

A   oral antibiotics
B   ciclosporin
C   acitretin
D   potent topical steroid
E   mild topical steroid.

**31** A 17-year-old girl presents with moderate acne vulgaris with exacerbations during menstruation. You suggest treatment with a combined oral contraceptive pill containing cyproterone acetate and ethinylestradiol, the patient has an excellent response. Which of the following skin conditions is also commonly exacerbated during menstruation:

A   oral lichen planus
B   psoriasis
C   lupus vulgaris
D   viral warts
E   herpes simplex infection.

**32** A 25-year-old man presents with an itchy rash on his elbows and knees. On examination he has a symmetrical rash consisting of excoriated grouped vesicles measuring a few millimetres in size. You perform a skin biopsy that shows fibrin and neutrophil accumulation at the tips of the dermal papillae. Direct immunofluorescence shows granular IgA deposition at the tips of the dermal papillae. Which of the following statements about this condition is true:

A   50% have gluten sensitive enteropathy
B   20% have a symptomatic gluten sensitive enteropathy
C   100% have an abnormal jejunal biopsy
D   80% have a symptomatic gluten sensitive enteropathy
E   20% have an abnormal jejunal biopsy.

**33** A 73-year-old patient presents with a number of intact blisters on the legs and torso. The blisters measure up to 6 cm in diameter and the patient describes a preceding pruritic eruption. A skin biopsy is performed that shows a sub-epidermal blister and IgG deposition at the basement membrane zone. Which of the following are not associated with this disorder:

A immunodeficiency
B diabetes
C HLA-DQ
D thyroid disease
E T-cell lymphoma.

**34** A 68-year-old woman presents with areas of oral ulceration and a widespread skin rash. She describes numerous thin blisters that appear on her skin and within her mouth and burst easily leaving raw erosions. A skin biopsy is taken and the patient is started on oral prednisolone 1 mg/kg/day. The skin biopsy shows subcorneal ulceration with prominent acantholysis. When the patient attends for review the prednisolone is not controlling the rash and it is decided to add in a second agent. Which of the following would not be appropriate:

A ciclosporin
B azathioprine
C cyclophosphamide
D mycophenolate mofetil
E oxytetracycline.

**35** A 30-year-old woman is referred by the obstetrics team with an itchy rash. She is in the third trimester of her first pregnancy. The patient describes a rash starting around her striae and spreading over much of her abdomen but sparing the umbilicus. On examination there is a mixture of urticated, erythematous plaques and papules on the abdomen with some excoriation. Blood tests have been undertaken by the obstetric team and show no abnormalities. What are the foetal and newborn risks for this woman's child:

A   small risk of miscarriage, no risk to newborn
B   small risk of miscarriage, moderate risk of newborn developing the rash
C   high risk of miscarriage, all newborns develop a transient rash
D   no risk to foetus, no risk to newborn
E   no risk to foetus, all newborns develop a transient rash.

**36** An 18-year-old girl presents as an emergency with a blistering rash, she is 33 weeks pregnant with her first child. She describes an abrupt onset of an itchy rash staring around the umbilicus and spreading. The next day numerous blisters started to appear from these itchy areas. On examination the patient has numerous intact blisters on an urticated base. She asks when the rash will resolve:

A   just prior to delivery
B   immediately post-delivery
C   a few weeks/months post-delivery
D   it will not resolve
E   it may resolve at any time prior to delivery.

**37** A 28-year-old woman is seen with known acne vulgaris. She has experienced an exacerbation of her acne since becoming pregnant. Which of these other skin complaints often worsens during pregnancy:

A   eczema
B   rosacea
C   plaque psoriasis
D   pityriasis rubra pilaris
E   lipomatosis.

**38** A 61-year-old man presents with a new rash. On examination there are large areas of hardened, indurated skin with nodules and plaques. On his right arm there is a flexion contracture due to the extensive skin involvement. He has a past history of hypertension related kidney failure. The patient feels that his skin problems started soon after having an MRI scan of his back. What is the most likely diagnosis:

A   morphea
B   nephrogenic systemic fibrosis
C   diabetic dermopathy
D   mycosis fungoides
E   systemic sclerosis.

**39** A 65-year-old woman presents with dyspareunia and pruritus of the vulva. On examination there are localised areas of white coloured thickening on the labia majora, labia minora and fourchette. There is partial resorption of the clitoris and some bruising. The patient has had no treatment, what would you recommend:

A   referral to a gynaecologist for surgery
B   tacrolimus (Protopic) ointment twice daily for 3 months
C   tapering dose of amitriptyline
D   clobetasone butyrate (Eumovate) cream daily for 2 months then taper
E   clobetasol (Dermovate) ointment daily for 1 month then taper.

**40** A 19-year-old man presents with an asymptomatic rash on the dorsum of his right hand. On examination there is an annular plaque with central clearing, the edge forms a ring of small skin coloured papules and the centre is slightly depressed. You suspect a solitary lesion of granuloma annulare. Which of the following is not a recognised treatment option in this scenario:

A   PUVA
B   no treatment
C   cryotherapy
D   potent topical steroids
E   photodynamic therapy.

## ANSWERS

### 21 C. Piebaldism

Vitiligo is a common, chronic disorder of depigmentation. It is more common in darker skin, young adults and those with a family history. It is strongly associated with other autoimmune conditions such as diabetes. Leukotrichia occurs when patches overlie hair bearing areas and koebnerization is seen after trauma. Treatment of vitiligo is unsatisfactory and usually comprises topical steroids, PUVA and cosmetic camouflage.

In this question pinta, leprosy, pityriasis alba and post-inflammatory patches from lupus are all acquired causes of hypopigmentation. Piebaldism is a rare inherited condition characterised by a white forelock and hypopigmented patches of skin, it is congenital not acquired.

Causes of acquired hypopigmentation:
- infection – leprosy, pinta, pityriasis versicolor
- post-inflammatory – scarring, lupus, eczema, pityriasis alba
- vitiligo
- halo naevus
- hydroquinones and other bleaching agents.

Causes of congenital hypopigmentation:
- piebaldism
- tuberous sclerosis
- naevus depigmentosus
- Waardenburg's syndrome.

### 22 B. Long term low dose aciclovir

The history given is typical for recurrent erythema multiforme (EM). EM occurs as a reaction to infection, medications or illness. It usually lasts for a few days then settles. Blisters may occur in the centre of the skin lesions and the mouth which may make it difficult to distinguish from the more serious Stevens-Johnson syndrome. It is more common in young adults and the rash has a predilection for the limbs.

Causes of erythema multiforme:
- infections (90%) – herpes simplex, orf, other viruses, mycoplasma, chlamydia, salmonella, tuberculosis, histoplasmosis, other fungi
- poison ivy, inflammatory bowel disease, lupus, Behçet's, pregnancy, radiotherapy
- non steroidal anti-inflammatory drugs, sulphonamides, anti-epileptic medications, antibiotics.

In this case the patient has developed recurrent EM following bouts of aphthous ulceration suggestive of herpes simplex infection. A long term low dose course of aciclovir is often helpful in this situation. Oral corticosteroids may be used to shorten the length and severity of acute episodes but in this case a short course of prednisolone would not prevent any recurrent episodes. IV immunoglobulins and ciclosporin are sometimes used to treat toxic epidermal necrolysis, they have no place in the treatment of EM.

## 23 E. Allopurinol

This patient has developed toxic epidermal necrolysis (TEN), a life threatening condition usually attributed to drug reactions. In TEN there is widespread keratinocyte death throughout the epidermis leading to large areas of skin loss. There is often a preceding fever and significant mucous membrane and eye involvement. TEN has 30–40% mortality, most often from sepsis, and those who survive often have long term ocular complications.

It is thought that Stevens-Johnson syndrome (SJS) and TEN are spectrums of the same disorder. There is however disagreement over whether erythema multiforme is also part of this spectrum. SJS may be caused by drug reactions, viral infections or malignancy but in up to 50% of cases no cause is found. The rash of SJS is similar to erythema multiforme with pronounced mucous membrane involvement. The treatment of SJS and TEN is supportive with some dermatologists advocating corticosteroids and intravenous immunoglobulins.

**Table 2.1** Key features of Stevens-Johnson syndrome (SJS) and toxic epidermal necrolysis (TEN)

| TEN | SJS |
| --- | --- |
| Severe skin pain | Little skin pain |
| Minimal mucous membrane involvement | Significant mucous membrane involvement |
| Diffuse erythema and skin loss | Targetoid skin lesions |
| Poor prognosis | Good prognosis |
| Greater than 30% skin involvement | Less than 10% skin involvement |

Common causes of toxic epidermal necrolysis:
- non-steroidal anti-inflammatory medications
- sulphonamides

- beta-lactam antibiotics
- anticonvulsants
- allopurinol.

In this question of the patient's medications allopurinol is the most likely to have precipitated the TEN.

## 24 B. Aspirin

Urticaria refers to weals or hives that appear on the skin due to a number of pathologies. The weals vary from a few millimetres to several centimetres in size, they are surrounded by a red flare and are often itchy. Urticaria may be accompanied by the deeper swelling of angioedema. Chronic ordinary urticaria is a common idiopathic illness resulting in multiple flares of urticaria for longer than six weeks. Although the cause is not known a number of medications and foods are known to exacerbate the condition.

Exacerbating factors in chronic ordinary urticaria:

- ACE inhibitors, aspirin, non-steroidal anti-inflammatory drugs, codeine
- caffeine, alcohol
- stress
- food additives e.g. benzoates, strawberries, tomatoes, fish, processed meat.

**Table 2.2** Subtypes of urticaria

| Type of urticaria | Features |
| --- | --- |
| Chronic ordinary urticaria | Idiopathic flares of an urticarial rash over many weeks, can be associated with autoimmune disorders and some patients have circulating autoantibodies |
| Acute ordinary urticaria | Can be due to a type 1 allergic response, also infection, serum sickness, non-allergic food reactions and non-allergic mast cell degranulators |
| Cholinergic urticaria | A physical urticaria, sweating leads to an urticarial rash |
| Cold urticaria | A physical urticaria, exposure to a cold temperature induces urticaria |
| Other physical urticarias | Other physical urticarias include delayed pressure, vibratory, localised heat, aquagenic, solar and exercise induced |
| Contact urticaria | This may be allergic – for example the proteins in a latex glove causing an IgE mediated degranulation of mast cells or non-allergic e.g. a nettle sting directly implanting histamine into the skin |

| Angioedema without urticaria | This may be an idiopathic phenomenon similar to chronic ordinary urticaria, ACE inhibitor related or due to C1 esterase inhibitor deficiency |
|---|---|
| Urticarial vasculitis | Weals that last longer than 24 hours and do not fully resolve and biopsy shows a vasculitis |
| Dermographism | A common form of physical urticaria, stimulation of the skin leads to an exaggerated triple response, often in young adults |

In this question aspirin is the most likely drug to have exacerbated the urticaria, doxepin and promethazine may be used to treat urticaria.

## 25 A. HIV test

This patient has ichthyosis acquisita an acquired disorder clinically and histologically similar to the congenital disorder ichthyosis vulgaris. It occurs in response to systemic disease most commonly Hodgkin's lymphoma.

Causes of ichthyosis acquisita:
- Hodgkin's lymphoma, mycosis fungoides, sarcomas and other internal malignancies
- AIDS, leprosy, tuberculosis, typhoid
- sarcoidosis
- hypothyroidism, panhypopituitarism
- nicotinic acid, butyrophenones, cimetidine.

In this case a HIV test would be useful to rule out AIDS a known cause of ichthyosis acquisita. The other tests suggested are not relevant to this diagnosis.

## 26 E. Wrist

Lichen simplex is a common dermatosis often seen in adult males. A stimulus such as an insect bite, patch of eczema or nervous habit leads to repetitive rubbing or scratching of an area of skin. Over time this patch of skin becomes thickened and pruritic initiating the itch-scratch cycle. Common sites for lichen simplex include the nape of the neck, shoulder, scalp, wrist, ankle and genitals. Treatment involves breaking the itch-scratch cycle with topical corticosteroids and a change in behaviour. In this question the wrist is another common site for lichen simplex to occur.

## 27 A. Sterile meningitis

This young patient is presenting with acne fulminans, the most severe form of cystic acne. It presents acutely in young men with a severe ulcerating acneiform rash and systemic upset.

Systemic features of acne fulminans:
- bone pain and osteolytic bone lesions commonly of the clavicle and sternum
- generalised systemic upset and fever
- hepatomegaly, splenomegaly, lymphadenopathy
- arthralgia, myalgia
- erythema nodosum.

Although often idiopathic acne fulminans may be precipitated by exogenous testosterone and isotretinoin. A rare serious complication, SAPHO syndrome, may occur in patients with acne fulminans.

Features of SAPHO syndrome:
- **S**ynovitis
- **A**cne – fulminans
- **P**ustulosis – pustules on the palms and soles
- **H**yperostosis
- **O**steitis.

Acne fulminans is treated with high dose antibiotics and/or systemic corticosteroids. In this question sterile meningitis is not a feature of acne fulminans.

## 28 C. Lithium

Acne may be caused by a number of medications and occupational exposures. Drug induced acne has a monomorphic appearance.

Causes of drug induced acne:
- corticosteroids, anabolic steroids, corticotrophin, ACTH
- phenytoin
- lithium
- isoniazid
- iodides – cold and asthma preparations
- bromide – sedatives and analgesics
- epidermal growth factor receptor inhibitors
- less often – azathioprine, ciclosporin, tetracyclines, vitamins, phenobarbital, psoralens.

Chloracne is an occupational dermatosis with patients developing small cystic papules and nodules following exposure to chlorinated hydrocarbons. Occupational acne may also be caused by insoluble substances that cause follicular occlusion such as oils, cosmetics and coal tars. Acne mechanica is another form of occupational acne where physical obstruction of follicles occurs by items such as helmets, collars and straps.

In this question lithium is the most likely responsible agent for his acne.

## 29 B. Northern European
Rosacea is a facial rash that affects the middle-aged and elderly. It is more common in women and those of Northern European and Celtic ancestry. It typically presents with erythema, telangiectasia, flushing, papules and pustules, more advanced disease may affect the eyes and the nose (rhinophyma). Rosacea is a multi-factorial disorder involving genetics and environment. The hair follicle mite demodex folliculorum and helicobacter pylori both seem to have a role in disease pathogenesis. Rosacea is worsened by steroids and treated with topical metronidazole and the oral antibiotics used in acne vulgaris.

**Table 2.3** Subtypes of rosacea

| Subtype of Rosacea | Clinical features |
| --- | --- |
| Erythematotelangiectatic | Prominent erythema and flushing, responds well to laser and pulsed light |
| Papulopustular | Papules and pustules predominate, may be mistaken for acne |
| Phymatous | Thickened skin leading to rhinophyma (nose), gnatophyma (chin) and metophyma (forehead). The eyelids, ears and cheeks may also be involved |
| Ocular | Irritated, red, dry and itchy eyes |
| Granulomatous | Large granulomatous nodules on the face |
| Pyoderma faciale | Severe disease with abrupt onset in young women |

In this question patients of Northern European ancestry are at higher risk of developing rosacea.

## 30 D. Potent topical steroid
This patient has a rash typical of lichen planus (LP) with oral and vulval involvement. LP tends to affect middle-aged adults although it is seen in all age groups. Patients present with a skin rash defined

by the '4 Ps' (pruritic, planar, purple, polygonal) papules, there are often lacy white streaks overlying the papules called Wickham's striae. Classical LP affects the skin and is commonly seen on the wrists, ankles and lower back, it tends to burn itself out in 12–18 months. Oral LP affects the inside of the cheeks and lateral tongue with painless white streaks or painful ulceration, it may be due to contact allergy to amalgam fillings. Genital LP may affect the vulva, vagina or penis leading to adhesions and ulceration. LP may also affect the hair (lichen planopilaris) and nails as discussed elsewhere in this book. Rare forms of LP include pigmented, actinic and bullous forms. Lichenoid drug reactions may occur and are often seen with gold, anti-malarial drugs and captopril. Clinicians should be alert to longstanding mucosal LP as it predisposes to squamous cell carcinoma.

In this question treatment is initially with potent or super-potent topical steroid. Second line agents include acitretin, ciclosporin and oral steroids.

## 31 E. Herpes simplex infection
Dermatological conditions showing menstrual exacerbation:
- acne vulgaris
- rosacea
- anogenital pruritus
- pityriasis capitis
- lupus
- eczema
- herpes simplex infections.

## 32 B. 20% have a symptomatic gluten sensitive enteropathy
This patient has a history and pathology consistent with dermatitis herpetiformis (DH), a chronic blistering skin condition with a predilection for the extensor surfaces. DH usually presents in young adults but it can affect patients of any age. It is characterised by very itchy vesicles that wax and wane in severity over time. There is a strong association between DH and gluten sensitive enteropathy (coeliac disease) which is present in 80–90% of patients although only 20% are symptomatic. Other autoimmune disorders such as thyroid disease are also strongly associated. Treatment is with a strict gluten free diet and dapsone. Longstanding, untreated disease has a potential risk of developing intestinal lymphoma.

## 33 A. Immunodeficiency

The history and pathological findings are typical of bullous pemphigoid a common immunobullous disorder of elderly patients. Patients develop a pruritic rash of erythematous patches and plaques that develop into thick-walled serous filled bullae. The blisters may spread all over the body and inside the mouth. Pathologically there are circulating autoimmune antibodies to the BP180/230 antigens contained within type XVII collagen. These target the hemidesmosomes at the basement membrane zone causing a dermal-epidermal split. Treatment is with corticosteroids and immunosuppressants with most cases burning out in 1–2 years. There is an association between bullous pemphigoid and other autoimmune disorders such as diabetes, HLA-DQ and certain T-cell lymphomas. Immunodeficiency does not predispose to bullous pemphigoid.

## 34 A. Ciclosporin

This patient has a history and histology consistent with pemphigus vulgaris a rare autoimmune bullous disorder. It presents with fragile superficial blisters of the skin and mucus membranes, in half of all patients the blistering is confined to the mouth. It often presents in late middle age and is more common in Jews and Indians. The blisters are superficial and do not scar but lesions may pigment. Pathologically there are circulating autoantibodies to desmoglein 3 a component of the desmosomes which attach keratinocyte cells together. Oral corticosteroids are considered first line therapy for pemphigus, second line agents include azathioprine, cyclophosphamide, mycophenolate mofetil, IVIG and rituximab.

**Table 2.4** Types of pemphigus

| Name | Clinical features |
|------|-------------------|
| Pemphigus vulgaris | Commonest, superficial blisters and erosions of the skin and mucosal surfaces |
| Pemphigus vegetans | Flaccid blisters are replaced by fungoid vegetations and pustules |
| Pemphigus foliaceus | Scaly crusted erosions with an erythematous base, no mucosal involvement |
| Pemphigus erythematosus | Similar to pemphigus foliaceus, photosensitive, may have positive ANA |

In this question ciclosporin would not be used as there is no evidence for effectiveness in pemphigus.

### 35 D. No risk to foetus, no risk to newborn

This patient is presenting with pruritic urticarial papules and plaques of pregnancy (PUPPP), the most common skin complaint of late pregnancy. Patients present with itchy, urticated papules and plaques staring in the striae and sparing the umbilicus. It is more common in primiparous ladies and does not tend to recur in future pregnancies. Treatment is with potent topical steroids and antihistamines. The rash resolves spontaneously and rapidly after delivery and there is no risk to the foetus or newborn.

### 36 C. A few weeks/months post-delivery

This patient has gestational pemphigoid which is also known as pemphigoid gestationis or herpes gestationis. It occurs in late pregnancy or immediately post-partum with an urticated pruritic rash that develops into vesiculobullae, rarely it may involve the mucosa. All patients have circulating anti-basement membrane zone autoantibodies and the histology and direct immunofluorescence are analogous to bullous pemphigoid. The rash often takes weeks to months to resolve post-delivery and there is a high risk of the rash developing in future pregnancies. The condition carriers a risk of premature delivery and small babies. In addition 10% of babies will develop the rash transiently after delivery. Treatment is with oral prednisolone.

**Table 2.5** Important rashes related to pregnancy

| Name | Foetal and newborn risk | Details |
|---|---|---|
| Gestational pemphigoid | Risk of premature labour, small babies and 10% newborns develop blisters | Abrupt onset of urticarial plaques and bullae in late pregnancy, recurs in future pregnancies, takes weeks-months to resolve post-partum, histologically similar to bullous pemphigoid, treat with oral steroids |
| Pruritic urticarial papules and plaques of pregnancy | Nil | Pruritic urticarial plaques and papules late in pregnancy, starts in abdominal striae, resolves post-partum, treat symptomatically |

| Prurigo of pregnancy | Nil | A diagnosis of exclusion, non-specific pruritus in mid/late pregnancy, treat symptomatically |
| Cholestasis of pregnancy | Risk of premature labour, meconium, foetal death, Vitamin K deficiency | Biochemical cholestasis leading to pruritus and frank jaundice, presents late, resolves on delivery, treat with ursodeoxycholic acid |

In this question the patient's gestational pemphigoid will settle within a few weeks to months post delivery.

### 37 B. Rosacea

A number of skin complaints tend to worsen during pregnancy, these include acne, rosacea, candidiasis and melasma. Some other skin conditions tend to improve in pregnancy such as eczema and psoriasis. Patients with pityriasis rubra pilaris are often treated with retinoids, this would be an absolute contraindication in pregnancy. Lipomatosis is not affected by pregnancy. A number of physiological changes may occur to the skin, hair and nails in pregnancy.

Physiological changes that may occur in pregnancy:
- hyperpigmentation - linea nigra, areola, melasma
- hair – hirsutism, frontal alopecia, telogen effluvium, androgenic alopecia
- nails – subungual hyperkeratosis, onycholysis, transverse grooving
- spider angiomas, varicosities, pyogenic granuloma
- palmar erythema
- oedema
- purpura
- gingival hyperplasia.

In this question rosacea tends to be exacerbated during pregnancy.

### 38 B. Nephrogenic systemic fibrosis

This patient is presenting with the recently described disorder nephrogenic systemic fibrosis (NSF) which is also known as nephrogenic fibrosing dermopathy. First described in 1997, patients present with progressive fibrosis of the skin and internal organs. NSF is seen in patients with renal failure who have been exposed to gadolinium contrast agents used in MRI scanning. As in this case patients develop nodules, plaques and large areas of indurated, hardened skin that can lead to flexion deformities. The histology of the skin lesions resembles scleroderma. The prognosis of NSF is uncertain with some patients having rapidly fatal fulminant disease and others showing complete resolution with time.

## 39 E. Clobetasol (Dermovate) ointment daily for 1 month, then taper

This patient is presenting with lichen sclerosus, an inflammatory dermatoses most commonly seen affecting the vulva of postmenopausal women. It presents with symptoms of dyspareunia, vulvodynia and pruritus. Thickened white patches occur on the vulva, perineal and perianal skin but the vagina itself is not affected. Bruises and haemorrhages may occur. Resorption of the clitoris, vaginal and urethral stenosis may also be seen. Treatment is initially with a tapering course of super-potent topical steroid, topical tacrolimus is used as a second line agent. Surgery may be needed for functional stenosis but fortunately this is rare. There is now good evidence that lichen sclerosus predisposes to vulval malignancy and patients should be made aware of this. Lichen sclerosus may also occur in prepubescent girls and men as detailed below.

**Table 2.6** Subtypes of lichen sclerosus

| Subtype | Clinical features |
| --- | --- |
| Adult female | Most common type, affects the vulva and perianal region, *see above* |
| Prepubescent female | May present in the vulval or perianal region, multiple ecchymoses are seen |
| Adult male | Affecting the foreskin, patients develop phimosis, painful erections and meatal stenosis |
| Prepubescent male | Rarely seen, may cause phimosis |
| Extragenital | Rough white patches of thickened skin are seen with or without associated genital disease, commonly on upper trunk, axillae and buttocks |

When vulval lichen sclerosus is seen in prepubescent girls the possibility of sexual abuse is often raised. Ecchymoses is a prominent feature of lichen sclerosus in this age group and inexperienced practitioners may erroneously attribute this to trauma. Sadly though child abuse does occur, and as lichen sclerosis koebnerizes this may be the presenting feature. Practitioners should treat each case with great care and sensitivity and request help from local experts as needed.

In this question appropriate first line treatment would be a tapering course of a super-potent topical steroid such as clobetasol.

## 40 A. PUVA

Granuloma annulare (GA) is a reasonably common skin disorder of young adults, although it may be seen in any age group. The history is often of relapsing and remitting skin lesions which heal without scarring. The rash may appear as a ring or red/skin coloured solitary lesions overlying joints. Localised disease is most common with one or a few lesions appearing in a similar anatomical site, it can though become more generalised. Generalised GA has been associated with diabetes, HIV and malignancy. Other rare forms include macular, erythematous, deep, actinic induced and perforating. A wide variety of treatments have been tried in GA which in itself is an indication that no one treatment is particularly efficacious. Treatments include topical, intralesional and systemic steroids, cryotherapy, photodynamic therapy, isotretinoin, methotrexate, dapsone and ciclosporin. PUVA is a well documented treatment in generalised GA but it would not be appropriate for a single lesion as in this case.

# Chapter 3
# Hair and nails

## QUESTIONS

**41** A patient presents with abnormal nails. On examination you see irregular coarse pitting of the nails with some transverse ridging. The also nails have a shiny appearance. What is the most likely cause:

A   lichen planus
B   eczema
C   Darier's disease
D   pachyonychia congenita
E   racket nails.

**42** You review a patient on the ward who had been admitted one month previously with a life threatening pneumonia. Examination of his nails shows a deep grooved transverse band approximately 3 mm from the cuticle. You suspect a diagnosis of Beau's lines. Which of the following is another cause of transverse grooves of the nail plate:

A   habit-tic dystrophy
B   lichen planus
C   racket nails
D   clubbing
E   argyria.

**43** A 23-year-old girl presents with abnormal spoon shaped nails; she has a past history of anaemia, dysmenorrhea and menorrhagia. You suspect a diagnosis of koilonychia. Which of the following is a recognised cause of koilonychia:

A macrocytic anaemia
B systemic lupus
C protein losing enteropathy
D lymphoedema
E liver cirrhosis.

**44** A young inpatient is referred for an opinion on her nails. She was admitted with suspected subacute bacterial endocarditis and splinter haemorrhages of the finger nails. A trans-oesophageal echocardiogram has been performed and shows no signs of valvular disease. Which of the following investigations is unnecessary:

A blood tests for rheumatoid factor and vasculitis screen
B review of her medications
C pregnancy test
D mantoux test
E occupational and social history taking.

**45** A 67-year-old patient presents with blue discolouration of their nails. Which of the following is the most likely cause:

A hydroxychloroquine
B renal failure
C tetracyclines
D gold injections
E heavy metal poisoning.

**46** A 44-year-old woman presents with a 6-month history of nail changes. On examination all 20 nails are abnormal with yellow discolouration and onycholysis. You suspect a diagnosis of yellow nail syndrome. Which of the following features is not known to be associated with this disorder:

A bronchiectasis
B recurrent sinus infections
C peripheral oedema
D pleural effusions
E flushing.

**47** A 19-year-old girl of Indian ethnicity presents to your clinic with a pigmented streak in her nail. She states that it has been present since she was a child but has recently darkened after a beach holiday in the Caribbean. On examination of her left thumb nail there is a darkly pigmented longitudinal streak that does not extend onto the proximal nail fold. What should you do:

A   reassure and discharge the patient
B   photograph the nail and review in three months time
C   perform a punch biopsy through the nail plate
D   perform a longitudinal nail biopsy
E   refer the patient for amputation of the distal thumb.

**48** A 14-year-old girl is referred with excessive hair. On examination she has a generalised increase in hair density and length over much of her body although her face is mostly spared. Which of the following is the most likely cause:

A   Turner's syndrome
B   prolactinoma
C   polycystic ovarian syndrome
D   anorexia nervosa
E   myotonic dystrophy.

**49** A 63-year-old woman is seen in clinic with psoriasis and appropriate treatment is initiated. She presents soon afterwards with generalised thinning of the hair. On examination there is no inflammation visible on the scalp and a forcible hair pluck reveals 40% of the hair in telogen. What is the most likely cause for the patient's hair loss:

A   no cause, normal hair
B   androgenic alopecia
C   alopecia areata
D   acitretin therapy
E   methotrexate therapy.

**50** An eight-year-old girl attends clinic with a 12-month history of hair loss. She denies any soreness or itching of the scalp and has no other rashes. On examination she has two well defined patches of hair loss on the crown and occipital scalp. The patches show non-inflamed, non-scarring alopecia with some exclamation mark hairs. Which of the following conditions has been associated with this condition:

A   acute myeloid leukaemia
B   atopy
C   HLA-B27
D   allergic contact dermatitis to hair products
E   tinea infection.

**51** You review a child with a widespread eczematous eruption and short fragile hair. Examination of the hair by light microscopy reveals hair that looks like bamboo with areas showing a ball-in-socket appearance. What is the most likely diagnosis:

A   Netherton's syndrome
B   trichothiodystrophy
C   monilethrix
D   trichorrhexis nodosa
E   pili torti.

**52** A 32-year-old Afro-Caribbean man presents to you with alopecia. He is known to the department with a past history of acne and hidradenitis suppurativa. On examination you see a scarring alopecia with fluctuant nodules, abscesses and sinus tracts. A biopsy shows inflammation and scarring with a predominantly neutrophilic infiltrate. What treatment would you recommend:

A   short course of flucloxacillin
B   excision and skin grafting
C   dapsone
D   isotretinoin
E   azathioprine.

**53** A middle-aged female patient presents with alopecia. On examination she has a multifocal scarring alopecia of the scalp with perifollicular erythema, pruritus and tenderness. She also has a non-scarring alopecia of the axillary and groin areas and a follicular keratotic rash. What is the most likely diagnosis:

A lupus
B Pseudopelade of Brocq
C Graham-Little syndrome
D keratosis follicularis spinulosa decalvans
E alopecia mucinosa.

# ANSWERS

## 41 B. Eczema

Although individually non-specific, the combination of coarse pitting, transverse ridging and shiny nails is typical of eczematous nail changes.

Table 3.1 Nail changes in inflammatory dermatoses

| Dermatoses | Nail changes |
|---|---|
| Lichen planus | Thin nail plate with longitudinal grooves and ridges (onychorrhexis), onycholysis, pterygium, complete loss of nails, can affect all the nails '20 nail dystrophy' |
| Eczema | Coarse pitting, transverse ridging, dystrophy, shiny nails |
| Alopecia areata | Fine pitting, rough nail surface, brittle nails |
| Darier's disease | Longitudinal ridges, triangular shaped 'nicks' at distal nail edge |
| Psoriasis | Pitting, nail thickening, onycholysis, brown discoloration, subungual hyperkeratosis, oil spots |

Table 3.2 Congenital disorders of the nail

| Disorder | Clinical features |
|---|---|
| Pachyonychia congenita | Thickened discoloured nails from birth, +/– keratoderma, keratin mutation |
| Racket nails | Common, autosomal dominant, broad short thumb nails |
| Nail-patella syndrome | Small poorly developed nails and knee caps, autosomal dominant |
| Congenital malalignment of the big toenails | Lateral deviation of the nail plate predisposing to ingrown toenails |
| Congenital hypertrophy of the lateral fold of the hallux | Rare, hypertrophy of the lateral nail fold in infants |
| Pincer nails | May be hereditary or acquired, over-curvature of the nail plate leading to severe pain |

## 42 A. Habit-tic dystrophy

Beau's lines are deep transverse grooves most often seen on the fingernails. They are due to a temporary cessation of cell division in the stem cells of the nail matrix commonly occurring in severe infection, they are also seen in localised trauma, chemotherapy use and systemic upset. Onychomadesis is proximal detachment of the nail – it has the same causes as Beau's lines. Argyria is systemic silver toxicity, it can affect the nail with the development of silver-grey lunulae.

In this question habit-tic dystrophy is another cause of transverse ridges and grooves. It is often associated with anxiety and often affects the thumb nails.

**Table 3.3** Patterns of nail plate abnormality and their associations

| Nail plate abnormality | Associated disorders |
| --- | --- |
| Pitting | Psoriasis, eczema, alopecia areata, lichen planus, Reiter's syndrome, incontinentia pigmenti |
| Transverse ridging | Beau's lines, eczema, psoriasis, habit-tic dystrophy, chronic paronychia, Raynaud's |
| Longitudinal ridging | Normal variant as age, lichen planus, Darier's disease |
| Onycholysis | Psoriasis, fungal infection, trauma, hyperthyroidism, cyanosis, Raynaud's, phototoxic reaction to tetracyclines, sarcoid, amyloid |

## 43 B. Systemic lupus

Koilonychia presents with thinned, flat nails with eversion of the lateral nail edges giving a spooned appearance. It is physiological in children, in adults is commonly due to iron deficiency anaemia.

**Table 3.4** Nail shape abnormalities and their associations

| Abnormality | Shape | Associations |
| --- | --- | --- |
| Koilonychia | Spoon shaped nails | Physiological in children, iron deficiency anaemia, trauma/occupation related, cachexia/deficiency of sulphur containing amino-acids, haemochromatosis, Raynaud's, lupus, congenital, diabetes |
| Leukonychia | White opaque nails | Hypoalbuminaemia, liver cirrhosis, malabsorption, malnutrition, congenital, trauma, keratoderma |
| Clubbing | Increased convexity of the nail fold, loss of the normal angle between the nail bed and fold | Inflammatory bowel disease, pulmonary neoplasms, lung fibrosis, bronchiectasis, bronchitis, liver cirrhosis, congenital heart disease, endocarditis, arteriovenous malformations, congenital |

## 44 D. Mantoux test

This young patient has presented with splinter haemorrhages of the finger nails and the admitting team have discounted the diagnosis of endocarditis. Distal splinter haemorrhages are common and often due to trauma, proximal splinters are rare and often due to systemic disease. Connective tissue disorders are a cause of proximal splinters along with the oral contraceptive pill and pregnancy. In this question active tuberculosis is not a known association and a mantoux test is not needed.

**Table 3.5** Other nail signs and their causes

| Disorder | Associations |
| --- | --- |
| Splinter haemorrhages | Subacute bacterial endocarditis, lupus, rheumatoid arthritis, vasculitis, antiphospholipid syndrome, malignancies, oral contraceptives, pregnancy, psoriasis, trauma, trichinosis, hypertension |
| Periungual erythema and nail fold telangiectasia | Rheumatoid arthritis, lupus, dermatomyositis, systemic sclerosis, Kawasaki's disease, Raynaud's, diabetes, mixed connective tissue disease |

## 45 A. Hydroxychloroquine

Discolouration of the nails may occur with a number of medications and localised or systemic illness. Blue discolouration is seen with quinines. Renal failure and gold can lead to brown discolouration. Heavy metal poisoning can lead to white transverse bands. Tetracyclines can stain nails yellow but can stain teeth blue-grey if given to the under-twelves.

**Table 3.6** Discolouration of the nails and associations

| Colour change | Associations |
| --- | --- |
| Blue | Cyanosis, anti-malarial drugs, haematoma, phenothiazines, Wilson's disease (lunula) |
| Blue-green | Pseudomonas infection (pyocyanin) |
| Black transverse bands | Cytotoxics |
| Brown | Fungal infection, nicotine staining, chloramphenicol, gold, Addison's disease |
| White spots | Trauma to nail matrix |
| White transverse bands | Heavy metal poisoning (Mee's lines) |
| White-brown | Chronic renal failure '50/50 nails' |

*continued*

**Table 3.6** *continued*

| Yellow | Psoriasis, fungal infection, jaundice, tetracyclines, lymphoedema, pleural effusion, immunodeficiency, bronchiectasis, sinusitis, rheumatoid arthritis, nephritic syndrome, thyroiditis, tuberculosis, Raynaud's |
|---|---|

## 46 E. Flushing

Yellow nail syndrome is a rare disorder that tends to present in middle-aged adults. Patients present with yellow-green discolouration of the nails, most pronounced at the lateral margins. The nails also thicken, nail growth slows and onycholysis may occur. It is associated with lymphoedema which may be of the extremities, face or genitals. 30% of patients develop pleural effusions, others develop recurrent bronchitis, chronic sinusitis or pneumonia. The disorder has also been associated with internal malignancy, immunodeficiency and rheumatoid arthritis. In yellow nail syndrome the changes are permanent and there is no effective treatment. Flushing is not a feature of the yellow nail syndrome.

## 47 A. Reassure and discharge the patient

In this question the patient is presenting with a longitudinal pigmented streak in her nail. The differential diagnosis of this is shown in Table 3.7.

**Table 3.7** Causes and features of pigmented streaks of the nail

| Cause of pigmented streak | Clinical features |
|---|---|
| Benign melanocytic naevus | Often longstanding the pigmented streak is uniform and may show pigmented bands |
| Epithelial melanin | Occurs in lentigo, racial pigmentation and drug induced pigmentation. It may affect multiple nails. The pigmented streak is homogeneous and may vary from light brown to dark gray |
| Malignant melanoma | New onset pigmentation of a single nail in an adult is concerning. The thumb and great toe nails are the commonest site for subungual melanoma. There is often irregularity of the pigment colour, spacing or thickness. Hutchinson's sign may be present with pigmentation spreading to the proximal nail fold |

In this case the patient has racial pigmentation and the nail streak is longstanding and has no suspicious features. Darkening of the pigmented streak in relation to recent sun exposure is not concerning. It would be reasonable to discharge the patient.

## 48 D. Anorexia nervosa

The history is consistent with hypertrichosis – an overgrowth of hair in a non-androgenic distribution. Hirsutism is excessive hair in a female occurring in a male (androgenic) pattern such as the beard and chest areas. In this question myotonic dystrophy is a cause of frontal hair loss; Turner's syndrome, prolactinoma and polycystic ovarian syndrome are causes of hirsutism. Anorexia nervosa is a cause of hypertrichosis.

Causes of hypertrichosis:
- congenital
- anorexia nervosa and other causes of malnutrition
- porphyria cutanea tarda
- dermatomyositis
- malignancy related
- minoxidil, phenytoin, ciclosporin, diaxoide, streptomycin, corticosteroids.

Causes of hirsutism:
- racial, idiopathic
- endocrine disturbance – acromegaly, prolactinoma, Cushing's syndrome, polycystic ovarian syndrome
- virilising tumours
- congenital adrenal hyperplasia
- exogenous androgens and oestrogens
- Turner's syndrome.

## 49 D. Acitretin therapy

This patient is presenting with generalised thinning of her hair with 40% of her hair in telogen, this is consistent with telogen effluvium. In a normal scalp 90–95% of hair will be in the anagen (growth) phase, a few hairs will be in catogen (transition) and 5–10% will be in telogen (shedding). A forcible hair pluck with over 15% of the hair in telogen is considered abnormal and is suggestive of telogen effluvium. The acute history does not fit with a diagnosis of androgenic alopecia or the patchy hair loss of alopecia areata. Telogen effluvium is often precipitated by a pathological or physiological change in health status.

In this question there is a causal link between initiating therapy for psoriasis and telogen effluvium occurring. Acitretin is a well documented trigger for telogen effluvium, methotrexate is a less frequently implicated drug.

Triggers for telogen effluvium:

- physiological shedding in newborns
- chronic/idiopathic form
- infection, illness, stress, post-partum, starvation, post-surgery
- endocrinopathies – Sheehan's syndrome, thyroid disease, parathyroid disease
- retinoids, other vitamin A derived drugs, anticoagulants, anti-thyroid drugs, anticonvulsants, heavy metals, beta blockers, chemotherapy, oral contraceptive pill.

## 50 B. Atopy

This child has a history and examination entirely consistent with alopecia areata. Often seen in children it presents with non-scarring patchy alopecia with a normal looking scalp and exclamation mark hairs. Although the pathogenesis is not fully understood it is a T-cell driven autoimmune disorder. Rarely, it may progress to total hair loss of the scalp (alopecia totalis) or loss of all hair on the body (alopecia universalis). In children the prognosis is good especially in limited disease; in adults and more advanced disease the prognosis is more guarded. Treatment includes corticosteroids, topical irritants and PUVA. Alopecia areata is associated with atopy, other autoimmune disorders and HLA-DQB1. Children with atopy and alopecia areata have a worse prognosis.

## 51 A. Netherton's syndrome

The description of bamboo-like hair with areas of a ball-in-socket appearance is characteristic of the hair shaft abnormality trichorrhexis invaginata. Netherton's syndrome is an autosomal recessive ichthyosis due to a mutation in the SPINK5 gene. It is characterised by short, spiky hair (trichorrhexis invaginata), multiple allergies and an ichthyotic rash with double edged scale (ichthyosis linearis circumflexa). It is also one of the commonest causes of erythroderma in a neonate.

**Table 3.8** Hair shaft abnormalities and their associations

| Name | Appearance | Associations |
|---|---|---|
| Trichorrhexis invaginata | Bamboo hair, ball-in-socket areas | Netherton's syndrome |
| Trichorrhexis nodosa | Split hair with frayed hairbrush-like ends | Either acquired secondary excessive straightening of hair or congenital where associated with mental retardation |
| Monilethrix | Elliptical nodules of normal hair thickness with areas of narrowing | Congenital, autosomal dominant, normal hair at birth, by a few months develop short brittle hair |
| Trichoschisis | Polarises with alternating light and dark bands | Sulphur deficient hair in trichothiodystrophy |
| Bubble hair | Large bubbles within hair shafts | Traumatic hair care, seen in young women |
| Pili torti | Flattened twisted hair shaft giving a spangled appearance | Can be part of ectodermal dysplasia with nail and dental abnormalities |
| Pili annulati | Air filled cavities within the hair shaft giving a ringed hair appearance | Congenital, autosomal dominant or sporadic |
| Trichonodosis | Knots occur in the hair | Gives a woolly appearance, can be associated with keratoderma and cardiomyopathy |
| Pili trianguli | Hair shaft has a triangular cross section | Spun-glass hair, difficult to comb |

## 52 D. Isotretinoin

In this question the patient is presenting with dissecting cellulitis of the scalp a rare condition which affects Afro-Caribbean males aged 20–40 years. It is a chronic condition with relapses and remissions that is strongly associated with severe acne and hidradenitis suppurativa. Treatment is challenging with isotretinoin often being the drug of choice.

Dissecting cellulitis of the scalp is in the group of primary neutrophilic scarring alopecias along with folliculitis decalvans also known as tufted folliculitis. In folliculitis decalvans a purulent folliculitis is seen with induration and bogginess of the scalp, it is often treated with antibiotics.

**Table 3.9** Causes of scarring alopecia

| Groupings | Causes |
|---|---|
| Biphasic alopecia | Longstanding non-scarring alopecia that with time scars e.g. androgenic alopecia, traction alopecia, alopecia areata |
| Primary neutrophilic scarring alopecia | Folliculitis decalvans, dissecting cellulitis of the scalp |
| Primary lymphocytic scarring alopecia | Lupus, lichen planopilaris, pseudopelade of Brocq, central centrifugal cicatricial alopecia, alopecia mucinosa, keratosis follicularis spinulosa decalvans |
| Secondary scarring alopecia | Direct destruction of the hair follicles e.g. burns, radiation, chronic infection, sarcoid, morphea |

## 53 C. Graham-Little syndrome

Graham-Little-Piccardi-Lasseur syndrome is a rare variant of lichen planopilaris and an example of a primary lymphocytic scarring alopecia. It presents with the triad of multifocal scarring alopecia of the scalp, non-scarring alopecia of the axillae and groin and a follicular lichenoid eruption on the body. It tends to present in middle-aged white women.

**Table 3.10** Causes and features of primary lymphocytic scarring alopecia

| Disorder | Clinical features |
|---|---|
| Lupus | The commonest cause. Well demarcated erythematous, scaly plaques leading to scarring, telangiectasia, dyspigmentation, hyperkeratosis and follicular plugging |
| Lichen planopilaris | Follicular lichen planus with hair shedding, pruritus, burning and tenderness. Seen in adult women it does not burn out like cutaneous disease; includes frontal fibrosing alopecia – progressive symmetrical recession of frontal hairline and Graham-Little syndrome – see above |
| Pseudopelade of Brocq | Multifocal flesh coloured patches of scarring alopecia 'footprints in the snow', it is slowly progressive eventually resolving spontaneously |
| Central centrifugal cicatricial alopecia | A descriptive term for a number of scarring alopecias that affect the vertex and crown of the scalp with a smooth and shiny, non-inflamed alopecia. Most commonly it occurs in Afro-Caribbean females due to chemicals and hot combs |

| | |
|---|---|
| Alopecia mucinosa | Rare follicular mucinosis of the scalp, 15% have underlying mycosis fungoides |
| Keratosis follicularis spinulosa decalvans | Widespread keratosis pilaris and scarring alopecia occurring in a child, it improves with puberty, can be congenital or spontaneous |

# Chapter 4

# Medical dermatology

## QUESTIONS

**54** A 30-year-old man presents to his family doctor with increased frequency of bowel motions, abdominal discomfort and weight loss. A colonoscopy is organised which shows changes consistent with active Crohn's disease. Inflammatory bowel disease may be associated with a number of cutaneous manifestations, which of the following is not a recognised association:

A   erythema nodosum
B   macular amyloidosis
C   pyoderma gangrenosum
D   angular cheilitis
E   small vessel vasculitis.

**55** You are asked to review a 76-year-old lady with longstanding rheumatoid arthritis. She has developed a number of painful haemorrhagic lesions on the finger pads. What is the most likely diagnosis:

A   Libman-Sacks endocarditis
B   drug reaction
C   Bywater's lesions
D   Janeway's lesions of subacute streptococcal endocarditis
E   Osler's nodes of subacute staphylococcal endocarditis.

**56** A 61-year-old Afro-Caribbean man presents with an itchy rash on his legs. The patient has a past medical history of longstanding diabetes and undergoes haemodialysis for diabetic related renal failure.

On examination he has a rash of multiple small papules with a central keratotic plug and excoriations. What is the most likely diagnosis:

A   perforating dermatosis
B   diabetic cheiropathy
C   rubeosis
D   acanthosis nigricans
E   diabetic dermopathy.

**57** A 34-year-old known alcoholic presents with severe abdominal pain radiating through to the back. Blood tests reveal a significantly raised serum amylase. On examination he has large ecchymosis-like lesions bilaterally on his flanks. What is the likely diagnosis:

A   pancreatic panniculitis
B   trauma related ecchymoses
C   Cullen's sign
D   Addison's related hyperpigmentation
E   Grey-Turner's sign.

**58** A 34-year-old woman presents to her family doctor with oligomenorrhea. Blood tests reveal a low free T4 and raised TSH. Which of the following cutaneous features occurs with this condition:

A   pretibial myxoedema
B   alopecia of the lateral third of the eyebrows
C   hyperhidrosis
D   thyroid acropachy
E   hyperpigmentation.

**59** You are asked to review a patient with a suspected basal cell carcinoma on his scalp. The patient is under the care of the hepatology team with longstanding hepatitis C infection and chronic liver failure. Whilst examining his skin which of the following features would you not expect to see:

A   palmar erythema
B   spider angiomas
C   hypopigmentation
D   gynaecomastia
E   loss of pubic hair.

**60** A patient is admitted under the general physicians with pneumonia. It is noticed that he has pronounced palmar erythema but no evidence of liver disease. On review the patient states that he has had red hands his whole life and his father has the same condition. Which of the following are not recognised causes of palmar erythema:

A   familial variant
B   pregnancy
C   hypothyroidism
D   leukaemia
E   systemic lupus.

**61** You are asked to review a 38-year-old woman on the renal unit who has been admitted with hypocalcaemia. What cutaneous feature would you expect to find:

A   erythroderma
B   calcinosis cutis
C   hair hypomelanosis
D   ridged, pigmented nails
E   widespread xeroderma with scale.

**62** A middle-aged patient presents with a 2-month history of acute onset flushing. She describes episodes where her face, neck and chest become acutely red. She has not been able to identify a particular precipitant. More recently during these episodes she becomes wheezy and develops diarrhoea. On examination telangiectasia are present in the distribution of the flushing and a cardiac murmur is heard. What is the investigation of choice for this patient:

A   transoesophageal echocardiogram
B   MRI of the adrenal glands
C   urine tests for 5-Hydroxyindoleacetic acid (5-HIAA)
D   thyroid function tests
E   urine tests for metanephrines.

**63** A 58-year-old man presents with generalised pruritus. On examination the skin shows only excoriations but widespread lymphadenopathy is also felt. Blood tests show a lymphocytosis with smear cells on the blood film. What is the most likely diagnosis:

A   acute lymphocytic leukaemia (ALL)
B   sarcoidosis
C   miliary tuberculosis
D   chronic myeloid leukaemia (CML)
E   chronic lymphocytic leukaemia (CLL).

**64** You see a 23-year-old man with excessive sweating. At rest in a cool room a starch iodine test is performed on the axillae that confirms the diagnosis of hyperhidrosis. Which of the following is not a cause of hyperhidrosis:

A   systemic sclerosis
B   acute infection
C   acromegaly
D   hypothalamic tumour
E   hyperthyroidism.

**65** A six-year-old girl presents with a chest infection and a high fever. The child has scanty hair growth, thin lightly pigmented skin and abnormal teeth. You suspect a diagnosis of anhidrotic ectodermal dysplasia. Which of the following is also a known cause of hypohidrosis:

A   hyperthyroidism
B   tricyclic antidepressants
C   hypoglycaemia
D   pregnancy
E   heavy metal poisoning.

**66** A 69-year-old patient presents to your clinic with suspected scabies. The patient describes a six month history of infestation with 'insects' the size a pen nib, he has been using malathion treatments weekly and says this offers some relief. On careful examination you see no evidence of infestation. The patient keeps pointing to hair follicles and small bits of fluff from his jumper saying these are the insects. Which of the pathologies listed below do you not need to consider in this patient:

A   cocaine abuse
B   scabies infestation
C   B12 deficiency
D   cerebrovascular disease
E   alcohol abuse.

**67** A 32-year-old man presents to A&E with bilateral painful legs and joint pains for a few days. On examination he has a number of tender subcutaneous nodules on the shins. Chest X-ray shows bilateral hilar lymphadenopathy, no other abnormalities are found on examination or baseline blood tests. What is the prognosis for this patient:

A   90% chance of complete resolution in the near future
B   90% chance of complete resolution but may take many years
C   50% chance of developing systemic disease
D   100% chance of developing systemic disease
E   no chance of developing systemic disease.

**68** A 42-year-old female lawyer presents with some lesions on her shins. The lesions are patches of shiny, red-brown skin with a yellow centre, in one area there is some early ulceration. You perform a biopsy which shows granulomas and necrobiosis consistent with necrobiosis lipoidica. After starting the patient on a super-potent topical steroid you organise for an overnight fasting glucose test which is reported as 5.8 mmol/L. The patient is upset as she has read on the internet that all people with necrobiosis lipodica have diabetes, what should you tell her:

A   she has diabetes
B   she has impaired glucose tolerance and is likely to develop diabetes in the future

C her test was normal but she definitely will develop diabetes in the future

D her test was normal but she has an increased risk of diabetes in the future

E her test was normal and she has no increased risk of developing diabetes.

69 A 48-year-old man presents with recurrent mouth ulcers. Which of the following is not a recognised cause of mouth ulceration:

A herpes simplex infection
B iron deficiency
C congenital syphilis
D nicorandil
E methotrexate in overdose.

70 A 58-year-old man presents with gynaecomastia. On examination he has symmetrical enlargement of both breasts with no evidence of any masses or suspicious lesions. The patient takes a number of medications and you suspect one may be responsible, which of the following is the most likely culprit:

A furosemide
B cimetidine
C ranitidine
D atorvastatin
E phenytoin.

71 A 92-year-old patient presents to the department with a patch of Bowen's disease. The patient has lifelong psoriasis and he remembers being treated with arsenic solution in the 1930s. What other cutaneous feature may you expect to see when examining the patient:

A Mee's lines in the nails
B periorbital oedema and hypopigmentation
C hyperkeratosis of the palms and soles
D a distinct dark halo in the iris
E superimposed guttate-like hyper and hypopigmentation.

**72** A 39-year-old man with longstanding active psoriasis presents with a number of petechiae and ecchymoses, in particular he has distinct purpura around his eyes. You suspect the patient has secondary systemic amyloidosis and perform a biopsy that confirms this. Which of the following conditions is not a recognised cause of amyloidosis:

A   multiple myeloma
B   pityriasis rosea
C   tuberculosis
D   rheumatoid arthritis
E   chronic myeloid leukaemia.

# ANSWERS

## 54 B. Macular amyloidosis

In this question macular amyloidosis is not a known cutaneous feature of inflammatory bowel disease. It is a primary amyloidosis of the skin presenting with reticular macular hyperpigmentation. Of note secondary systemic amyloid may be associated with longstanding inflammatory bowel disease and presents with petechiae and ecchymoses.

Cutaneous manifestations of inflammatory bowel disease:
- erythema nodosum, erythema multiforme
- pyoderma gangrenosum, Sweet's syndrome, other neutrophilic dermatoses
- small vessel vasculitis, cutaneous polyarteritis nodosa
- fistulae and abscesses in perianal region
- pruritus ani, vulvi and scrota
- acquired acrodermatitis enteropathica.

Oral associations with inflammatory bowel disease:
- aphthous ulcers
- granulomatous cheilitis, angular cheilitis
- gingival/mucosal swelling
- cobblestoning of buccal mucosa.

## 55 C. Bywater's lesions

The description and history in this question is consistent with Bywater's lesions a cutaneous manifestation of rheumatoid arthritis. They are cutaneous infarcts related to small vessel rheumatoid vasculitis. In addition they may also present under the nails as painless red-brown lesions mimicking the splinter haemorrhages of subacute bacterial endocarditis (SBE). Libman-Sacks endocarditis is a sterile endocarditis which occurs in patients with systemic lupus. Osler's nodes are painful, red, raised lesions on the palms and soles which may be associated with SBE. Janeway's lesions are small asymptomatic maculo-nodules on the palms or soles and are pathognomonic of SBE.

Rheumatoid arthritis has a large number of cutaneous manifestations including:
- neutrophilic dermatoses – pyoderma gangrenosum, rheumatoid neutrophilic dermatoses, Sweet's syndrome, neutrophilic panniculitis
- palisading granulomas – rheumatoid nodules and papules,

palisaded neutrophilic and granulomatous dermatitis, interstitial granulomatous dermatitis
- vascular – small, medium and large vessel vasculitis, capillaritis, Bywater's lesions
- purpura
- palmar erythema
- thin skin
- drug reactions to therapies.

## 56 A. Perforating dermatosis
This patient is likely to have a perforating dermatosis also known as Kyrle's disease, a rare cutaneous manifestation of diabetes. The rash is most commonly seen in Afro-Caribbean patients on dialysis for diabetic related renal failure. It is characterised by itchy papules with a keratotic plug on the extensor surface of the legs. It is difficult to treat and topical retinoic acid is often tried.

Cutaneous features of diabetes:
- infections – candidal, fungal, bacterial, gangrene
- necrobiosis lipoidica diabeticorum
- acanthosis nigricans – velvety hyperpigmented patches in axillae
- diabetic dermopathy – brown atrophic macules on the legs
- diabetic thick skin
- diabetic bullae – tense, non-inflammatory, often on legs
- yellow-orange skin – carotenaemia
- diabetic ulcers
- perforating dermatosis
- eruptive xanthomas
- acral erythema – erysipelas-like erythema of hands and feet
- diabetic cheiropathy – thickened skin, reduced joint movement, contractures
- disseminated granuloma annulare
- rubeosis – chronic flushed appearance of face, neck and chest.

## 57 E. Grey-Turner's sign
In this question the patient is presenting with Grey-Turner's sign – bilateral bruising of the flanks. This is a cutaneous sign of acute haemorrhagic pancreatitis and carriers a grave prognosis. Other causes of Grey-Turner's sign include blunt abdominal trauma, ruptured aortic aneurysm and ruptured ectopic pregnancy.

Cutaneous features of pancreatitis:

- Grey-Turner's sign
- Cullen's sign – black-blue bruising around the umbilicus
- pancreatic panniculitis – tender, fluctuant nodules on the lower legs
- jaundice
- livedo reticularis
- urticaria
- thrombophlebitis migrans – pancreatic malignancy associated.

## 58 B. Alopecia of the lateral third of the eyebrows
This patient is presenting with a cutaneous feature of hypothyroidism – alopecia of the lateral third of the eyebrows. All the other signs in this question including pretibial myxoedema occur in thyrotoxicosis.
Cutaneous features of hypothyroidism:
- dry, rough, course, cold, pale skin with a boggy/oedematous feel yellow discolouration
- hypohidrosis
- acquired ichthyosis, palmoplantar keratoderma
- tuberous xanthomas
- dull, course, brittle hair, diffuse alopecia, alopecia of the lateral third of eyebrows
- thin, brittle, striated nails with slow growth, onycholysis.

Cutaneous features of hyperthyroidism:
- fine, velvety, smooth skin which is warm and moist to the touch
- hyperhidrosis
- localised or generalised hyperpigmentation (raised adreno-corticotropic hormone (ACTH))
- palmar erythema
- pretibial myxoedema
- fine, thin hair, mild diffuse alopecia
- onycholysis, koilonychia, thyroid acropachy.

## 59 C. Hypopigmentation
There are a number of cutaneous features of chronic liver disease including hyperpigmentation. In this question hypopigmentation is not a feature.
Cutaneous features of chronic liver disease:
- clubbing of the nails, leukonychia
- palmar erythema
- spider angiomas
- diffuse pigmentation

- loss of axillary and pubic hair
- gynaecomastia
- xanthelasma if obstructive element.

## 60 C. Hypothyroidism

Palmar erythema is a non-specific sign that may occur in a number of conditions. It can also be a familial variant inherited in an autosomal dominant manner. In this question hyperthyroidism is a cause of palmar erythema, hypothyroidism is not.

Causes of palmar erythema:
- familial variant
- chronic liver disease, alcohol abuse
- pregnancy
- connective tissue disorders e.g. lupus, rheumatoid arthritis, sarcoid
- thyrotoxicosis
- polycythaemia
- leukaemia
- inflammatory dermatoses e.g. eczema, psoriasis, erythroderma
- chemotherapy, anti-epileptic medications
- HTLV1 infection
- paraneoplastic – especially brain malignancies.

## 61 E. Widespread xeroderma with scale

The cutaneous features of hypocalcaemia are rarely seen except in advanced renal disease. Patients present with a number of features including widespread xeroderma and scale. In this question hypocalcaemia is not a cause of erythroderma, calcinosis cutis, hair hypomelanosis or pigmentation of the nails. Cutaneous features respond to treatment with calciferol therapy.

Cutaneous features of hypocalcaemia:
- widespread xeroderma with scale
- loss of body hair
- fragile, broken nails with secondary candidal infection
- impetigo herpetiformis – grouped pustules on an erythematous base, often associated with pregnancy.

## 62 C. Urine tests for 5-Hydroxyindoleacetic acid (5-HIAA)

This patient has acute onset of flushing associated with bronchospasm, diarrhoea and a cardiac murmur, this is suggestive of carcinoid syndrome. Carcinoid syndrome occurs when a neuroendocrine carcinoid tumour metastasises to the liver and releases serotonin and other mediators into the blood stream. Patients may also develop a pellagra-like photodistributed skin rash and the flushed areas may have a violaceous hue. Carcinoid syndrome is investigated by testing urine for metabolites such as 5-HIAA. In this question the history is not typical for a phaeochromocytoma.

Causes of facial flushing:
- physiological, abrupt cessation of exercise, emotional or sexual arousal
- menopausal
- carcinoid syndrome
- phaeochromocytoma
- autonomic dysfunction, migraine, neurological lesions
- systemic mastocytosis
- hyperthyroidism
- neoplasms.

Drug related flushing:
- ACE inhibitors
- calcium channel blockers
- alcohol
- nitrates
- opioids
- calcitronin.

## 63 E. Chronic lymphocytic leukaemia (CLL)

In this question the patient is presenting with generalised pruritus, lymphadenopathy, lymphocytosis and smear cells; the most likely diagnosis is CLL. ALL is rare in adults and a lymphocytosis would not be seen in CML. Sarcoidosis and miliary tuberculosis are both causes of widespread lymphadenopathy but the blood picture does not fit with these conditions. Generalised pruritus may be caused by a number of pathologically significant medical conditions and all patients should be thoroughly investigated.

Medical causes of generalised pruritus:
- iron, B12 or folate deficiency
- hyperthyroidism, hypothyroidism
- liver diseases
- malignancy
- HIV related
- haematological – leukaemia, lymphoma, polycythemia, myeloma

- drug reactions
- renal failure (late sign)
- recreational drug abuse
- psychogenic, neuropathic.

## 64 A. Systemic sclerosis

The commonest cause of hyperhidrosis is primary or idiopathic hyperhidrosis which tends to occur after puberty in patients with a strong family history. There is excessive sweating of the axillae, palms and soles during waking hours. Acute infection, acromegaly, hypothalamic tumours and hyperthyroidism are all causes of hyperhidrosis. In this question systemic sclerosis causes hypohidrosis due to physical destruction of the sweat glands.

Causes of hyperhidrosis:
- primary, idiopathic, familial (majority)
- acute infection
- endocrine disturbance – acromegaly, hyperthyroidism, hypoglycaemia, menopause, pregnancy
- primary neurological lesions of the hypothalamus, pons, medulla or spinal cord
- degenerative neurological conditions affecting the autonomic nervous system
- drugs – alcohol, opioids, mercury, arsenic
- vasomotor – heart failure, Raynaud's syndrome, connective tissue disorders
- compensatory hyperhidrosis.

## 65 B. Tricyclic antidepressants

Hypohidrosis is a potentially life threatening condition due to hyperpyrexia. In this question hyperthyroidism, hypoglycaemia, pregnancy and heavy metal poisoning are all causes of hyperhidrosis. Tricyclic antidepressants cause a reversible hypohidrosis due to their anticholinergic effects.

Causes of hypohidrosis:
- primary neurological lesions of the hypothalamus, pons, medulla or spinal cord
- degenerative neurological conditions affecting the autonomic nervous system
- congenital insensitivity to pain with anhidrosis
- peripheral neuropathies – diabetes, leprosy, amyloid, alcohol

- hypohidrotic ectodermal dysplasias
- local destruction of sweat glands – systemic sclerosis, tumours, burns, radiation
- obstruction to sweat glands – miliaria, ichthyosis, psoriasis
- skin of premature infants
- drugs – tricyclic antidepressants, oxybutinin, phenothiazines.

## 66 B. Scabies infestation

In this question the patient is suffering from delusional parasitosis, a form of psychosis where patients develop a false delusional belief that they are infested with parasites or insects. In this case the patient is highly unlikely to have scabies as he can see the 'insects' (scabies mites cannot be seen with the naked eye) and has had repetitive treatments with malathion. Delusional parasitosis may be a primary psychosis or secondary to a number of pathologies that should be excluded.

Pathologies that may induce delusional parasitosis:
- cocaine, alcohol, amphetamines and other drugs of abuse
- B12 deficiency
- cerebrovascular disease and other neurological disorders
- hypothyroidism
- neoplasms
- diabetes.

Treatment of delusional parasitosis is with antipsychotics and the prognosis is poor.

## 67 A. 90% chance of complete resolution in the near future

In this question the patient is presenting with Löfgren's syndrome, an acute presentation of sarcoidosis. Patients have a triad of erythema nodosum, arthralgia and bilateral hilar lymphadenopathy. They may also have a fever. This is a transient disorder in which 90% of patients have complete resolution within two years, a small number of patients may go on to develop systemic sarcoidosis.

Causes of erythema nodosum:
- idiopathic
- Löfgren's syndrome, systemic sarcoidosis
- inflammatory bowel disease
- drugs – oestrogens, sulphonamides, penicillins, bromides, iodides
- infections – yersinia, salmonella, campylobacter, respiratory viral infections, brucellosis, mycoplasma, tuberculosis, histoplasmosis, hepatitis B

- neutrophilic dermatoses
- pregnancy
- malignancy related, especially haematological malignancies.

## 68 D. Her test was normal but she has an increased risk of diabetes in the future

This patient has a history and pathology consistent with necrobiosis lipoidica. Although the rash is commonly seen on the shins it may appear elsewhere on the body. Starting as a painless non-specific papule it breaks down into a raised red-brown patch with a central yellow colour and telangiectasia, atrophy and ulceration may follow as the lesion matures. Necrobiosis lipoidica is more common in women and tends to present in early middle age. Sixty per cent of patients with necrobiosis lipoidica have frank diabetes of the other 40% some have impaired glucose tolerance and the rest are at increased risk of diabetes in the future. In this question the patient has an upper normal fasting glucose and may develop diabetes in the future.

**Table 4.1** Interpretation of overnight fasting glucose test results

| Glucose | Relevance |
| --- | --- |
| 3.6 to 6.0 mmol/L | Normal |
| 6.1 to 6.9 mmol/L | Impaired glucose tolerance |
| 7.0 mmol/L or above | Probable diabetes |

## 69 C. Congenital syphilis

Causes of mouth ulceration:
- aphthous, idiopathic
- traumatic
- herpes simplex infection
- B12 deficiency, iron deficiency
- coeliac disease, inflammatory bowel disease
- Reiter's syndrome
- immunodeficiency
- nicorandil, methotrexate, chemotherapy
- oral cancers, metastatic cancer
- syphilitic snail track ulcers
- inflammatory dermatosis e.g. pemphigus.

In this question congenital syphilis is not a cause of mouth ulceration, although secondary syphilis is.

**70 B. Cimetidine**

Gynaecomastia in a male is often due to an imbalance of the oestrogens and androgens. Unilateral gynaecomastia is suspicious of underlying malignancy and should be investigated thoroughly. Obesity may cause a pseudo-gynaecomastia due to adipose tissue deposition.

Causes of gynaecomastia:

- puberty related
- hypogonadism – Klinefelter's syndrome, testicular failure
- liver cirrhosis, alcohol abuse, other liver disease
- hyperthyroidism
- malnutrition
- tumours – adrenal, testicular, lung, pancreas, gastrointestinal, liver
- drugs – spironolactone, digoxin, oestrogens, cimetidine, steroids, cannabis.

In this question cimetidine is the most likely cause of the patient's gynaecomastia.

**71 E. Superimposed guttate-like hyper and hypopigmentation**

Arsenic solutions were used to treat a variety of illnesses including psoriasis until the 1940s. Disorders of hyper and hypopigmentation are a common long term complication from arsenic ingestion. Mee's lines are a sign of acute arsenic or heavy metal poisoning presenting a few months after the episode and growing out over 1–2 years. The other suggested presentations are not a feature of chronic arsenic toxicity.

Acute features of arsenic toxicity:

- flushing, erythema, facial oedema, urticaria
- alopecia, Mee's lines, loss of nails
- gastrointestinal upset, neuropathy, pancytopenia, cardiac arrhythmias, renal failure, respiratory failure.

Chronic features of arsenic toxicity:

- hyperpigmentation of the axillae, groin, nipples, palms, soles, pressure points
- superimposed 'raindrop' pattern of guttate hypo and hyperpigmentation
- alopecia
- arsenic keratosis – premalignant papules on the palms and soles
- skin cancers, other cancers.

## 72 B. Pityriasis rosea

Amyloid is an extracellular deposit made of fibril proteins, glycosaminoglycans and lipoproteins. The composition of the amyloid fibril protein depends on its precursor protein and is related to the type of amyloidosis and the clinical presentation.

**Table 4.2** Types of amyloidosis

| Type | Derivation | Clinical features |
|---|---|---|
| Systemic amyloid | May be primary (AL fibril protein), myeloma related (AL) or secondary (AA) | 30% have skin lesions such as petechiae, ecchymoses, pinch purpura, periocular purpura, papules, nodules and plaques, also have mucous membrane and systemic involvement – macroglossia, hepatomegaly, splenomegaly, lymphadenopathy, cardiac, renal and neurological disease |
| Lichen amyloid | Keratinocyte tonofilament derived fibril protein | Flesh coloured brown papules with scale which may coalesce into plaques, limited to cutaneous involvement, more common in men from the Middle East, Asia and South America |
| Macular amyloid | Keratinocyte tonofilament derived fibril protein | Pruritic macular rippled hyperpigmentation common on the back and neck, limited to cutaneous involvement, more common in men from the Middle East, Asia and South America |
| Nodular amyloid | AL fibril protein | Solitary or multiple waxy nodules on the face, scalp, legs or genitals, histologically indistinguishable from systemic amyloid, 15% of patients develop systemic amyloid |

Secondary systemic amyloidosis may occur in patients with longstanding inflammatory, infectious or malignant conditions such as myeloma, tuberculosis, rheumatoid arthritis and leukaemia. In this question pityriasis rosea is a short lived eruption and is not associated with amyloidosis.

# Chapter 5

# Collagen-vascular disorders and immunology

## QUESTIONS

**73** A 22-year-old woman is referred to your clinic with nail changes. On examination she has finger pulp atrophy, telangiectasia of the nail folds and generalised thinning of the nails with longitudinal ridging. You suspect the patient may have Raynaud's disease. If this is the case what pattern of colour change would you expect to see in the fingers when the patient is exposed to a cold environment then warmed:

A cyanosis → pallor → erythema
B erythema → cyanosis → pallor
C cyanosis → erythema → pallor
D pallor → erythema → cyanosis
E pallor → cyanosis → erythema.

**74** You are referred a 50-year-old man with a photodistributed rash and muscle weakness. On examination the rash has a violaceous hue with areas of hypo and hyperpigmentation, telangiectasia and epidermal atrophy consistent with poikiloderma. On closer examination the patient also has a distinctive heliotrope rash around the eyes and thickened skin over the knuckles. Which of the following blood tests will help with your diagnosis:

A erythrocyte sedimentation rate
B creatine kinase
C C-reactive protein
D anti-neutrophilic cytoplasmic antibodies (ANCA)
E anti-Scl 70 antibodies.

**75** You are asked to see a 19-year-old man referred by his family doctor with a suspected diagnosis of plantar pustular psoriasis. When you see him he is quite upset as he has been ill for some time and 'no one knows what is wrong with me!' Two months ago he went on holiday with a group of friends to a European resort known for its exuberant nightlife. Soon after returning he felt generally unwell with episodic swelling of his knee and ankle joints and red, sore eyes. Despite repeated courses of antibiotics and eye drops his symptoms have not improved. Recently he developed a rash on the soles of his feet consisting of hard, tender lumps, scaly patches and pustules. He has no nail changes and does not smoke. What is the likely diagnosis:

A subacute bacterial endocarditis (SBE)
B psoriasis with psoriatic arthropathy
C Behçet's syndrome
D Reiter's syndrome
E systemic lupus.

**76** A 25-year-old man of Greek descent is referred to your clinic with suspected erythema nodosum. He gives a long history of general illness, throat infections, muscle and joint pains, weight loss, headache and malaise. More recently he has developed painful ulcers on his penis and inside his mouth and red swollen eyes. In the patient's antecubital fossa a small ulcer is present where a blood test was taken the previous week. Which of the following skin lesions are not associated with this syndrome:

A   necrobiosis lipoidica
B   sterile papulopustules
C   erythema nodosum
D   Sweet's-like neutrophilic dermatosis
E   pyoderma gangrenosum.

77 An eight-year-old girl presents four days after suffering a coryzal illness. She has subsequently developed palpable purpura on her legs and buttocks, arthralgia and colicky abdominal pain. Her blood pressure is normal and urine dipstick has 1+ blood and 1+ protein. What is the appropriate course of action:

A   discharge the patient with reassurance
B   admit the patient for dialysis
C   start a course of oral prednisolone and follow her up in clinic
D   admit the patient for intravenous cyclophosphamide
E   organise a 24-hour urinary protein and blood pressure measurements.

78 A 52-year-old woman presents to clinic with livedo reticularis. On examination she also has tender small subcutaneous lumps on her legs and an early ulcer on her left shin. You perform a skin biopsy which shows a panarteritis consistent with vasculitis. You carefully examine the patient and can find no signs of systemic involvement; the patient feels well in herself and denies any weight loss. She has normal blood pressure, a clear urine dipstick and a negative serum ANCA blood test. What is the most likely diagnosis:

A   Henoch-Schönlein purpura
B   polyarteritis nodosa
C   cutaneous polyarteritis nodosa
D   microscopic polyangiitis
E   Churg-Strauss syndrome.

**79** A 25-year-old woman presents with some cosmetically disfiguring plaques on her abdomen. On examination she has three large thickened scar-like patches of skin with a slight mauve discolouration. The skin is shiny, hairless and smooth with no obvious sweating. Which of the following is not a known precipitant of this disorder:

A   cocaine abuse
B   borrelia infection
C   pregnancy
D   measles infection
E   a recent burn injury.

**80** You are asked to review a patient with known systemic sclerosis and worsening Raynaud's phenomenon. During the consultation the patient mentions a new symptom of progressive shortness of breath on exertion. What would be the most appropriate investigation:

A   peak expiratory flow reading
B   a sputum sample for microbiology and mycology
C   high resolution CT scan of the chest
D   staging CT scan of the chest
E   left sided cardiac catheterisation.

**81** A 42-year-old man presents with an asymmetrical polyarthritis, mouth ulcers and abnormal nails. The arthritis is mostly confined to the distal interphalangeal (DIP) joints. Nail changes include pitting and oil spots. Blood tests reveal an elevated ESR and negative rheumatoid factor. There is no cutaneous evidence of psoriasis, although the patient does have a family history. What is the likely diagnosis:

A   psoriatic arthritis
B   seronegative rheumatoid arthritis
C   osteoarthritis
D   gonococcal arthritis
E   pseudogout.

**82** An 18-year-old man with known Crohn's disease is referred due to persistent ulceration around his ileostomy site. A biopsy of the ulcer has shown a diffuse neutrophilic infiltrate and marked tissue necrosis, gram staining was negative. Prior treatment with topical betamethasone valerate had little benefit. Which of the following treatment options would be least appropriate:

A   oral corticosteroids
B   infliximab
C   ciclosporin
D   topical clobetasone butyrate
E   dapsone.

**83** You review a 70-year-old lady referred with an ulcer on her leg. On examination there is a 7 cm shallow ulcer overlying the medial malleolus with surrounding haemosiderin deposition and mild pitting oedema. The ulcer has been present and slowly enlarging over the past 12 months. What is the most appropriate course of action:

A   punch biopsy and referral for radiotherapy
B   arterial dopplers and refer to a vascular surgeon
C   arterial dopplers and compression therapy
D   swab the ulcer and start antibiotics
E   incisional biopsy and start corticosteroids.

**84** You are asked to review an infant on the paediatric ward with a rash on their legs. On examination the child has a net-like reddish-blue rash comprised of dilated capillaries and surrounding pale central areas. The child is well in themselves and the mum says that the rash occurred for the first time when they went for a walk on a chilly winter's day. What is the likely diagnosis:

A   erythema ab igne
B   cutis marmorata
C   cutaneous polyarteritis nodosa
D   cutis marmorata telangiectatica congenita
E   idiopathic livedo reticularis.

**85** A 13-year-old girl presents with tender red-purple papules on the tips of her fingers and toes. She says that these have occurred every winter, starting itchy and then becoming tender. Her family doctor has sent some blood tests that were unremarkable. How should you proceed:

A   advise keeping the extremities warm +/- a topical steroid
B   admit for a prostaglandin infusion
C   start mepacrine
D   perform an incisional biopsy
E   refer for angiogram and vascular studies.

**86** You are asked to review an inpatient with myelofibrosis and a rash, the admitting team are concerned about vasculitis. On examination of the distal limbs there is a non-blanching rash consisting of multiple 1–2 mm diameter flat red-purple lesions. What is the likely diagnosis:

A   microscopic polyangiitis
B   thrombocytopenia related petechiae
C   polyarteritis nodosa
D   meningococcal septicaemia
E   vitamin K deficiency.

**87** A 52-year-old man is seen with a rash on his legs. On examination the rash is composed of multiple palpable 5–10 mm purple lesions which do not blanch. The patient is systemically unwell with fever, haematuria and mouth ulceration. Which diagnosis is the least likely:

A   disseminated intravascular coagulation
B   lupus related vasculitis
C   microscopic polyangiitis
D   pneumococcal septicaemia
E   rheumatoid arthritis related vasculitis.

**88** A middle-aged woman of African descent is seen with a red-brown plaque on her right cheek. Biopsy shows caseating epithelioid granulomas without surrounding lymphocytes. Blood tests show a raised erythrocyte sedimentation rate and an isolated raised calcium. What is the most likely diagnosis:

A   systemic lupus
B   tuberculosis
C   granuloma faciale
D   subacute lupus
E   sarcoidosis.

**89** You see a patient with chronic scarring alopecia. On examination they also have fixed, indurated, erythematous papules and plaques on the face and ears. There are also areas of scarring, hyperpigmentation and hypopigmentation. On the scalp there is scale and keratotic plugging of the hair follicles. You suspect a diagnosis of discoid lupus, what is the chance of this patient developing systemic lupus:

A   100% by 10 years
B   100% by 6 months
C   50%
D   5%
E   none.

**90** You are referred a patient with suspected drug induced lupus. Blood tests have shown positive single stranded DNA, ANA and anti-histone antibodies. Which of the following medications is the likely culprit:

A   ramipril
B   methotrexate
C   simvastatin
D   loperamide
E   phenytoin.

**91** What pattern of autoantibodies would you expect to see in a patient with advanced systemic lupus including lupus nephritis and neurolupus:

A   peripheral ANA, dsDNA, Anti-SCL 70, Anti-La
B   speckled ANA, ssDNA, Anti-RNP, Anti-Ro
C   homogenous ANA, dsDNA, Anti-sm, Anti-RNP
D   centromeric ANA, dsDNA, Anti-SCL 70, Anti-La
E   nucleolar ANA, ssDNA, Anti-centromere, Anti Jo-1.

**92** You are asked for advice by a family doctor who has an 83-year-old patient with an extensive rash. He feels that the patient may have an autoimmune bullous disorder and he has sent a serum immunology screen which has shown a positive c-ANCA. What is the most likely diagnosis:

A   pemphigus vulgaris
B   bullous pemphigoid
C   linear IgA disease
D   dermatitis herpetiformis
E   epidermolysis bullosa acquisita.

**93** An 82-year-old man presents with a 4-week history of a rash. He described an initial rash of highly pruritic erythematous plaques which developed into blisters. On examination he has a number of intact blisters measuring 2–15 cm in size over his extremities and trunk, there is no mucous membrane involvement. You suspect a diagnosis of bullous pemphigoid and organise for an incisional biopsy and blood tests. What pattern of direct immunofluorescence (IMF) would you expect to see:

A   intraepidermal IgG
B   linear IgA on the basement membrane zone (BMZ)
C   intraepidermal IgA and C3
D   linear IgG and C3 on the BMZ
E   granular IgA and C3 on the BMZ.

**94** (Continued from question 93.) What pattern of indirect immunofluorescence would you expect to see:

A   IgG anti-BMZ antibodies
B   IgG anti-epidermal antibodies
C   IgA anti-BMZ antibodies
D   IgA anti-epidermal antibodies
E   IgM anti-BMZ antibodies.

**95** You are asked to see a woman who is 36 weeks pregnant on the antenatal ward. On examination she has a number of thick-walled, intact blisters predominantly on the abdomen. You suspect a diagnosis of gestational pemphigoid and perform a biopsy for histology and IMF. Direct IMF shows linear deposition of C3 and IgG along the basement membrane zone. What antigen is the IgG targeting:

A Desmoglein 1
B Desmoglein 3
C plectin
D BP antigen 2 (BP 180)
E type VII dermal collagen.

**96** A 12-year-old boy presents with a palpable purpuric rash on his legs and buttocks, he also gives a history of joint pains and abdominal discomfort. If you were to biopsy the rash and perform direct IMF what pattern of immune complex deposition would you expect to see:

A IgM and C3 around deep vessels
B IgA around superficial and deep vessels
C IgG on the BMZ and around vessels
D fibrinogen around superficial vessels
E IgG around superficial and deep vessels.

## ANSWERS

### 73 E. Pallor → cyanosis → erythema

Raynaud's phenomenon is a vasospastic disorder affecting the fingers and less commonly the toes. Triggers such as cold or emotional distress cause vasospasm in the digits. Longstanding Raynaud's phenomenon leads to ischaemic changes in the digits such as pulp atrophy, thin brittle nails, nail fold telangiectasia and ulceration. Treatment includes avoiding triggers (cold) and vasodilating drugs such as nifedipine and prostaglandins. Raynaud's phenomenon may either be a primary disorder or secondary to a number of different pathologies:

Raynaud's phenomenon as part of a connective-tissue disorder:
- scleroderma, CREST syndrome
- systemic lupus
- dermatomyositis, polymyositis
- rheumatoid arthritis.

Raynaud's phenomenon due to impeded vascular supply:
- atherosclerosis
- Buerger's disease
- thoracic outlet syndrome.

Drug causes of Raynaud's phenomenon:
- cytotoxic medications
- beta blockers
- ciclosporin
- vinyl chloride (occupational exposure)
- heavy metals.

Other:
- vibration related
- haematological disorders such as cryoglobulinaemia
- reflex sympathetic dystrophy.

In this question the colour changes in Raynaud's phenomenon are of pallor (white) leading to cyanosis (blue) and finally erythema (red).

### 74 B. Creatine kinase

This middle-aged patient is presenting with dermatomyositis. Patients present with a photodistributed rash and a proximal extensor myopathy which may extend with muscles becoming tender. There is a bimodal distribution with juvenile form associated with calcinosis cutis and an adult form which may be associated with malignancy. Systemic manifestations include malaise, arthritis, cardiac disease and pulmonary fibrosis.

Cutaneous manifestations of dermatomyositis:
- photodistributed violaceous poikilodermic rash which may be plaque-like on the extensors and over the knuckle pads (Gottron's papules)
- a light purple (heliotropic) rash around the eyes
- cuticle nail fold dystrophy and telangiectasia
- periorbital oedema
- calcinosis cutis – childhood form only.

The myositis releases muscle enzymes into the blood and these are measured as increased levels in creatine kinase, LDH and aldolase. Dermatomyositis may also be ANA positive, ANCA is negative as are anti-Scl 70 antibodies – a marker of scleroderma. Treatment of dermatomyositis is with systemic steroids and immunosuppressants.

## 75 D. Reiter's syndrome
In this question the young man is presenting with a reactive arthritis, also known as Reiter's syndrome. Given the preceding history of travel it is likely to have been precipitated by either a chlamydial infection or enteric infection such as salmonella, shigella or campylobacter. Eighty per cent of patients who develop Reiter's syndrome have the haplotype HLA-B27.

Clinical features of Reiter's syndrome:
- arthritis – self limiting, intermittent, worse lower limbs
- urethritis – may be severe in men and asymptomatic in women
- ocular inflammation – conjunctivitis, uveitis
- psoriasiform skin lesions.

Patients may also develop oral ulceration and are at increased risk of developing deep vein thrombosis (DVT).

Cutaneous manifestations of Reiter's syndrome:
- keratoderma blennorrhagicum – occurs after 1–2 months, hard, tender lumps, scaly patches and pustules on soles of feet
- circinate balanitis – rash on the head of the penis
- other psoriasiform-like skin lesions.

The patient has no heart murmur characteristic of SBE and the skin lesions are described as psoriasiform rather than vasculitic. Behçet's syndrome is characterised by recurrent oral and genital ulceration not present in the case. The rash is also not typical for lupus. Psoriasis remains a possibility with the signs of a pustular rash, arthritis and conjunctivitis but the lack of nail changes and rapid onset of symptoms is more suggestive of Reiter's syndrome.

## 76 A. Necrobiosis lipoidica

This patient has many features consistent with Behçet's syndrome a multisystem polysymptomatic disorder which is often difficult to diagnose. The disorder it more common in groups from the Mediterranean, Middle East and Far East, often presenting in males aged 20–30 years.

Clinical features of Behçet's syndrome:
- prodrome of general illness, can be for many years
- recurrent, painful, genital and oral ulceration which may extend throughout the GI tract
- ocular inflammation, such as uveitis
- skin lesions
- pathergy
- neurological involvement, which may be fatal.

Cutaneous features of Behçet's syndrome:
- erythema nodosum is common
- acne-like sores on the limbs and trunk
- sterile papulopustules
- Sweet's-like neutrophilic dermatosis
- pyoderma gangrenosum
- palpable purpura/vasculitis.

In this question necrobiosis lipoidica is not a feature of Behçet's syndrome but is classical of the distinct disorder necrobiosis lipoidica diabeticorum.

## 77 E. Organise a 24-hour urinary protein and blood pressure measurements

This patient is presenting with the classical tetrad of Henoch-Schönlein purpura (HSP):
- rash – symmetrical palpable purpura commonly on the legs and buttocks
- arthritis – transient polyarthritis of lower limbs
- abdominal pain – colicky, may have diarrhoea or colonic bleeding
- kidney impairment.

HSP is a form of leukocytoclastic vasculitis, most often seen in children under the age of 10 years. It is often preceded by a coryzal illness attributed to beta-haemolytic streptococci, although a variety of drugs and other infections have also been implicated. Mild self-limiting kidney involvement is seen in up to half of all cases but only 1–5% progress to end-stage renal failure.

Most patients do not require treatment as HSP is a self limiting condition. It is though prudent to organise for urine and blood pressure testing to pick up the small number of patients who develop long term renal problems. In this question the patient has only mild renal involvement and does not need active treatment or admission to hospital.

## 78 C. Cutaneous polyarteritis nodosa

In this question the patient is presenting a vasculitis limited to the skin with no evidence of systemic involvement. Given the panarteritis nature of the vasculitis on biopsy this is consistent with cutaneous polyarteritis nodosa (PAN). Cutaneous PAN is a rare vasculitis of small and medium sized arteries affecting the skin and subcutaneous tissues, it tends to run a chronic and benign course. It is important to distinguish it from the potentially life threatening systemic PAN which involves the skin and other tissues such as the liver, kidney, gastrointestinal tract, nervous system and lungs. Cutaneous PAN is treated with corticosteroids and immunosuppressants, patients need to be followed up carefully as a small number progress to systemic PAN.

Cutaneous signs of vasculitis:
- purpura, petechiae, papules and nodules
- livedo reticularis
- ulcers and ulcerative lesions
- urticaria
- Raynaud's phenomenon
- haemorrhagic blisters
- pyoderma gangrenosum.

All the other potential answers to this question represent systemic vasculitides which would not fit with the description.

**Table 5.1** Summary of systemic vasculitides and their features

| Vasculitis | Vessels involved | Features |
| --- | --- | --- |
| Giant cell (temporal) arteritis | Large | A granulomatous vasculitis affecting the aorta and its branches, a predilection for the temporal artery can lead to blindness if untreated |
| Takayasu's arteritis | Large | A granulomatous vasculitis affecting the aorta and its branches leading to stenosis, thrombosis and aneurysms |
| Kawasaki disease | Medium | Predominantly affecting children this vasculitis presents with lymphadenopathy, glossitis, cheilitis and conjunctivitis, if untreated serious cardiac involvement may occur |
| Churg-Strauss syndrome | Medium and small | An eosinophilic vasculitis with a predilection for the lungs, gastrointestinal system and nerves |
| Polyarteritis nodosa | Medium and small | A multisystem necrotising vasculitis which may be fatal |
| Microscopic polyangiitis | Small | A multisystem necrotising vasculitis that may mimic PAN or systemic lupus |
| Wegener's granulomatosis | Small | A multisystem vasculitis with a predilection for the upper airways, eyes and ears, difficult to distinguish from Churg-Strauss |

## 79 A. Cocaine abuse

This patient is presenting with skin plaques typical of morphea also known as localised scleroderma. Morphea may affect adults and children with typical plaques of shiny, hairless thickened skin. It most commonly affects the trunk but if a limb is affected by large plaques of morphea it may lead to muscle wasting and stiffness. Over many years the plaques tend to soften leaving hyperpigmentation and depressed scars.

Although in most cases there is no identified precipitant, it can follow:
- borrelia infection (Lyme disease)
- pregnancy
- measles and other viral infections
- localised injury or trauma
- other autoimmune disorders such as lichen sclerosus.

**Table 5.2** Subtypes of morphea

| Type of morphea | Clinical features |
| --- | --- |
| Plaque morphea | Commonest type, oval plaques 1–20 cm of thickened scar-like skin, lilac coloured edge |
| Superficial morphea | Symmetrical patches seen in the groin, axillae and under the breasts |
| Linear scleroderma | A linear streak of morphea seen on a limb in a child |
| Generalised morphea | Rare, widespread morphea-like change |
| En coup de sabre | Deep seated morphea of the scalp and temple, scarring alopecia, bone changes |

In this question there is no known association between recreational drug use such as cocaine and morphea.

## 80 C. High resolution CT scan of the chest

Systemic sclerosis is a multisystem autoimmune connective tissue disorder of unknown cause. It is more common in women and most commonly presents in early middle age.

Cutaneous features of systemic sclerosis:

- Raynaud's phenomenon – often the presenting feature, *see* question 73
- symmetrical hardening of the skin on the fingers and face that may generalise, the skin is thickened, telangiectatic and has hypo and hyperpigmentation
- fragile nails with dilated nail fold capillaries and periungual erythema
- sclerodactyly – resorption of the finger tips
- ulcers
- calcinosis.

Systemic features of systemic sclerosis:

- gastrointestinal – oesophageal dysmotility, reflux, small bowel disease, colonic diverticulum
- renal – progressive renal failure and hypertension
- cardiorespiratory – lung fibrosis, cardiomegaly, pulmonary hypertension
- joints – arthralgia, tendon rupture, proximal muscle weakness.

Systemic sclerosis presents with a spectrum of severity which may be reflected in the autoimmune antibody profile.

**Table 5.3** Key features of limited and generalised systemic sclerosis

| Type | Features | Antibody profile |
| --- | --- | --- |
| Limited systemic sclerosis | Skin changes limited to hands and face | ANA, anti-centromere |
| Generalised systemic sclerosis | Organ and widespread skin involvement | ANA, SCL-70 |

CREST syndrome is a form a limited systemic sclerosis characterised by Calcinosis, Raynaud's phenomenon, oEsophageal involvement, Sclerodactyly and Telangiectasia.

In this question the most likely cause of the patient's shortness of breath is lung fibrosis, an often fatal manifestation of systemic sclerosis. The investigation of choice for interstitial lung disease is a high resolution CT scan. Pulmonary hypertension is another possible cause of progressive shortness of breath in systemic sclerosis and this could be investigated with a right sided cardiac catheterisation.

## 81 A. Psoriatic arthritis
Psoriatic arthritis occurs in up to 30% of patients with psoriasis, in 15% of these patients the arthritis may precede the development of the rash. In this question the patient has nail changes typical of psoriasis and a family history of psoriasis. The distribution of the arthritis in the DIP joints is also typical of psoriatic arthritis. Osteoarthritis which may also occur in the DIP joints would be unusual in the patient of this age.

**Table 5.4** Patterns of psoriatic arthritis

| Pattern | Clinical features |
| --- | --- |
| Asymmetrical mono/ oligoarthritis | Commonest presentation, predilection for the DIP's and proximal interphalangeal (PIP) joints |
| DIP arthritis | Arthritis confined to the DIP's, strongly associated with psoriatic nail changes |
| Rheumatoid arthritis like | Arthritis in a rheumatoid-like pattern but often seronegative |
| Arthritis mutilans | Rare, destructive arthritis leading to telescoping of the fingers |
| Spondylitis and sacroiliitis | Resembling ankylosing spondylitis, the knees may also be involved |

## 82 D. Topical clobetasone butyrate

This young patient is presenting peristomal ulceration typical of pyoderma gangrenosum (PG). Crohn's disease is a well described risk factor for PG and the neutrophilic infiltrate on biopsy is typical. PG often starts as a tender pustule or papule and breaks down into a sharply defined ulcer with violaceous undermined edges.

Conditions associated with pyoderma gangrenosum:

- inflammatory bowel disease
- most inflammatory arthritis, vasculitic and connective tissue disorders
- haematological paraproteinaemias and malignancies
- Sweet's syndrome and other neutrophilic dermatosis.

The treatment of PG is immunosuppression, either locally with topical steroids or with systemic agents such as ciclosporin and methotrexate. Anti-inflammatory medications such as dapsone and tetracyclines have also been used with variable success. In this question a potent topical steroid, betamethasone valerate (Betnovate), has been tried with little effect and there would be little to gain by swapping to a medium potency topical steroid such as clobetasone butyrate (Eumovate).

## 83 C. Arterial dopplers and compression therapy

In this question the patient has a typical venous ulcer; it is large and shallow and overlies the medial malleolus. There is other evidence of venous insufficiency with haemosiderin deposition and pitting oedema. Venous ulceration is treated with compression and dressings, arterial dopplers are needed prior to compression therapy to check that the arterial supply is not compromised. The case history is not typical of a malignancy or other type of leg ulceration.

**Table 5.5** Characteristics of leg ulcers

| Type of ulcer | Clinical features |
|---|---|
| Venous ulceration | Often large, shallow ulcers with an irregular, ill-defined border on the lower leg and ankle. Associated with haemosiderin deposition, oedema, varicosities, atrophie blanche, lipodermatosclerosis, stasis dermatitis and subcutaneous calcification |
| Pro-coagulant ulcers | Similar to venous ulcers but smaller. Occur in haematological disorders such as sickle cell disease, hereditary spherocytosis and anterior tibial syndrome<br>*continued* |

**Table 5.5** *continued*

| | |
|---|---|
| Arterial ulcers | Round, sharply demarcated ulcers in distal sites and over bony prominences. Associated with hairless, shiny atrophic skin, claudication, poor peripheral pulses, reduced capillary refill, cold feet and thickened toenails |
| Neuropathic (trophic) ulcers | Distal ulceration overlying pressure sites associated with reduced sensation. Occurs in a number of neurological disorders including diabetes, leprosy, tabes dorsalis, porphyria, amyloid, nerve injury and spinal pathology |
| Pressure ulcers | Ulcers overlying bony prominences in immobile patients, commonly on the sacrum, hips and malleoli |
| Vasculitic ulcers | Occur over dependant areas and are often painful, associated with cutaneous vasculitic rashes |
| Pyoderma gangrenosum | *See* question 82 |
| Infective ulcers | Rare, a number of causes including brucellosis, leprosy, leishmaniasis and atypical mycobacterium |

## 84 B. Cutis marmorata

This case describes a reticulated (net like) vascular rash occurring on the legs of a child consistent with livedo reticularis. Primary livedo reticularis may present as cutis marmorata, cutis marmorata telangiectatica congenita or idiopathic livedo reticularis. Cutis marmorata is described in the question, it occurs in 50% of infants as a physiological response to cold, the rash is asymptomatic, mild and transient. Cutis marmorata telangiectatica congenita is rare, it presents after birth with a severe livedo associated with congenital abnormalities. Idiopathic livedo reticularis occurs in young women in response to the cold, with repeated attacks the rash may become permanent. Livedo reticularis may also occur as a secondary phenomenon to other underlying disorders.

Causes of secondary livedo reticularis:

* vasculitis, inflammatory arthritis and connective tissue disorders
* haematological abnormalities – cryoglobulinaemia, antiphospholipid syndrome, polycythaemia, thrombocytosis, pro-clotting disorders
* embolic
* chronic infections such as tuberculosis
* malignancies.

Erythema ab igne is another reticulated rash which occurs in response to a thermal or radiation injury to the skin. It is classically seen on the legs of elderly patients with hypothyroidism who sit too close to an electric fire. Another commonly seen presentation is on the abdomen of young girls who have been using a hot water bottle for prolonged periods of menstruation pains.

Although polyarteritis nodosa is a rare cause of livedo reticularis it would be highly unusual in an infant and there are no other symptoms or signs of a vasculitis.

## 85 A. Advise keeping the extremities warm +/- a topical steroid

In this question the patient is presenting with chilblains, also known as pernio or perniosis. Chilblains are a localised form of vasculitis precipitated by cold exposure. In young patients it tends to occur in the winter for a few seasons then settles, the prognosis is more guarded in the elderly. Treatment is difficult and consists of avoiding the cold, topical steroids and not smoking.

The differential diagnosis includes chilblain lupus, which is rare in the young and cold sensitive blood dyscrasias which may be screened for. There is no indication for a biopsy or vascular studies in this patient.

## 86 B. Thrombocytopenia related petechiae

The rash described consists of flat red-purple macules less than 4 mm in diameter, this is a macular petechial rash. The commonest causes of petechial rashes are platelet problems, in this case thrombocytopenia related to myelofibrosis.

Causes of a macular petechial rash:
- thrombocytopenia and its multitude of causes
- abnormal platelet function disorders
- valsalva-like pressure to the skin e.g. blood pressure cuff
- scurvy
- venous eczema
- pigmented purpuric eruptions e.g. Schamberg's.

Macular purpura are larger flat red-purple lesions with a diameter of 5–9 mm. They commonly occur in patients with a background platelet problem and acute inflammation or infection. Both primary vasculitis and sepsis related vasculitis tend to present with palpable purpura, vitamin K deficiency results in ecchymoses.

## 87 A. Disseminated intravascular coagulation

This patient is presenting with a palpable purpuric rash, the classical rash of a vasculitis. Commonly there is prominent erythema around the rash and on occasions it may break down into an ulcer.

Causes of a palpable purpuric rash:
- primary vasculitides
- immune complex related vasculitis – idiopathic, sepsis related, drug associated, secondary to connective tissue disorders
- non-vasculitic – erythema multiforme, PLEVA, pigmented purpuric eruptions.

In this question disseminated intravascular coagulation is the least likely diagnosis, it tends to present with ecchymoses or macular petechiae not palpable purpura.

Ecchymoses are flat round-oval purpuric lesions often over 1 cm in size, they normally result from minor trauma on a background of dermal fragility, platelet dysfunction or an anticoagulated state.

## 88 E. Sarcoidosis

In the question the woman is presenting with features of sarcoidosis a systemic granulomatous disorder of unknown aetiology. It is more common in people of Afro-Caribbean descent and women. It is histologically characterised by caseating epithelioid granulomas. Chronic sarcoidosis should be distinguished from Löfgren's syndrome – an acute transient sarcoid associated with erythema nodosum. Three patterns of cutaneous sarcoid are seen, often with overlap.

**Table 5.6** Patterns of cutaneous sarcoid

| Type of cutaneous sarcoid | Clinical features |
| --- | --- |
| Cutaneous sarcoid | Non-scarring red-brown plaques on the face, upper back and extremities; scarring alopecia |
| Lupus pernio | Violaceous plaques on the nose, ears or cheeks which blanch to an apple jelly appearance, tends to scar, strongly associated with sarcoidosis of the lungs |
| Darier-Roussy | Painless, firm, mobile subcutaneous nodules |

Systemic features of sarcoidosis:
- lung fibrosis
- bone cysts
- iritis, uveitis

- hypercalcaemia, calcium renal stones
- hepatomegaly, splenomegaly, lymphadenopathy
- pituitary infiltration, panhypopituitarism, diabetes insipidus
- neurosarcoid, mononeuritis multiplex – especially facial nerve palsy
- scarring alopecia
- arthritis, arthralgia.

## 89 D. 5%

This patient has the typical signs of discoid lupus (DLE), a chronic photoexacerbated autoimmune disorder. In answer to the question approximately 5% of patients with DLE will go on to develop systemic lupus (SLE); although around 25% with SLE will develop DLE-like skin lesions. DLE is treated with topical steroids, anti-malarial drugs, photoprotection and in resistant cases immunosuppression.

**Table 5.7** Subtypes of cutaneous lupus

| Subtype | Clinical features |
|---|---|
| Discoid lupus | The commonest eruption, scaly patches/plaques on the head and neck with scarring alopecia, ~5% develop SLE |
| Subacute lupus | A strikingly photosensitive rash occurring on the back and chest, often annular, associated with Anti-Ro, ~25% develop SLE |
| Acute cutaneous lupus | A transient photosensitive butterfly rash on the face, strongly associated with SLE |
| Lupus tumidus | A photosensitive dermal rash, often annular and urticated, similar to Jessner's lymphocytic infiltrate |
| Lupus profundus | Lupus panniculitis occurs clinically as firm, deep nodules that heal as cosmetically disfiguring indurated scars |
| Neonatal lupus | Children born to mothers with systemic lupus may develop a transient annular rash, these children should be assessed for congenital heart block |
| Chilblain lupus | Chilblains, nail fold telangiectasia, may also have Raynaud's phenomenon |
| Rowell's syndrome | A combination of cutaneous lupus and erythema multiforme, may be severe |
| Systemic lupus | Photosensitive butterfly rash, non-specific erythematous eruptions, periungual erythema, nail fold telangiectasia, DLE-like rash, alopecia, subcutaneous nodules, leg ulcers, purpura, livedo reticularis, chilblain lupus, urticaria, erythema multiforme, pigmentary changes |

Systemic features of SLE:
- polyarthritis, arthralgia
- pleurisy, pleural effusions
- pericarditis, valvular lesions
- lupus nephritis
- lymphadenopathy, splenomegaly
- retinal lesions
- neurolupus, peripheral neuropathy.

## 90 E. Phenytoin

Susceptible individuals are at risk of developing a drug induced lupus. Patients present with a chronic history of musculoskeletal problems (arthritis, myalgia, arthralgia) and serositis (pleurisy, pericarditis), cutaneous manifestations are rarely seen. Serum immunology is positive for single stranded DNA, ANA and anti-histone antibodies. Treatment is withdrawal of the offending medication.

Common causes of drug induced lupus:
- procainamide
- hydralazine
- isoniazid
- chlorpromazine
- anticonvulsants including phenytoin
- methyldopa
- minocycline
- lithium.

A drug induced lupus syndrome may also occur when using anti-TNF medications, this tends to present with cutaneous manifestations and a positive double stranded DNA antibody. A number of mediations may also induce subacute lupus.

Medications that may induce subacute lupus:
- hydrochlorothiazide
- terbinafine, griseofulvin
- calcium channel blockers
- non steroidal anti-inflammatory drugs
- antihistamines.

In this question phenytoin is the most likely drug to have caused drug induced lupus.

## 91 C. Homogenous ANA, dsDNA, Anti-sm, Anti-RNP

Anti-nuclear antibodies (ANA) are autoantibodies directed against the contents of the cell nucleus. An ANA of greater than 1:40 is considered to be significant, although 15% of people over the age of 55 years have a positive ANA. The test is reasonably sensitive but poorly specific with a large number of autoimmune disorders showing a positive result. The pattern of ANA seen can be associated with certain conditions:

**Table 5.8** Patterns of anti-nuclear antibody and their relevance

| ANA pattern | Association |
|---|---|
| Homogenous pattern | Suggestive of lupus |
| Peripheral/rim pattern | Suggestive of lupus |
| Speckled pattern | Suggestive of mixed connective tissue disease |
| Centromeric pattern | Specific for limited systemic sclerosis |
| Nucleolar pattern | Suggestive of systemic sclerosis |

Extractable nuclear antigens (ENA) are more specific nuclear autoantibodies which can be helpful in the diagnosis of connective tissue disorders.

**Table 5.9** Extractable nuclear antigens and their associations

| ENA | Association |
|---|---|
| Anti-Ro (SS-A) | Sjögren's syndrome, subacute lupus, SLE, foetal heart block |
| Anti-La (SS-B) | Sjögren's syndrome, subacute lupus, SLE |
| Anti-sm (smith) | Specific marker for SLE |
| Anti-dsDNA | Specific for lupus, lupus nephritis |
| Anti-ssDNA | Drug induced lupus, rheumatoid arthritis, myositis, systemic sclerosis |
| Anti-RNP | Most connective tissues disorders, mixed connective tissue disease, neurolupus |
| Anti-Scl 70 | Systemic sclerosis |
| Anti-centromere | Limited systemic sclerosis, CREST syndrome |
| Anti-Jo1 | Myositis |

In this question an autoantibody pattern of homogenous ANA, dsDNA, Anti-sm and Anti-RNP is most likely to be seen in a patient with advanced SLE with kidney and neurological involvement.

## 92 A. Pemphigus vulgaris

Anti-neutrophilic cytoplasmic antibodies (ANCA) are a group of autoantibodies targeted against the cytoplasm of neutrophils and monocytes. They are most commonly used as a marker for systemic vasculitis but are also positive in a number of other autoimmune disorders.

**Table 5.10** Anti-neutrophilic cytoplasmic antibodies and their associations

| ANCA | Target protein | Associations |
| --- | --- | --- |
| p-ANCA | Myeloperoxidase | Microscopic polyangiitis, Churg-Strauss syndrome, ulcerative colitis |
| c-ANCA | Proteinase 3 | Wegener's granulomatosis, pemphigus vulgaris |

Another commonly used autoantibody is rheumatoid factor (RF) an antibody which targets the Fc portion of IgG molecules. RF is a sensitive marker for rheumatoid arthritis and Sjögren's syndrome with high levels associated with extra articular disease. It may also be positive in other connective tissue disorders, chronic hepatitis, chronic infections and haematological malignancies.

In this question the patient has an immunobullous disorder and positive C-ANCA, this would be consistent with pemphigus vulgaris.

## 93 D. Linear IgG and C3 on the BMZ
## 94 A. IgG anti-BMZ antibodies

Direct and indirect immunofluorescence (IMF) are useful and sometimes crucial tools in the diagnosis of immunobullous disorders.

**Table 5.11** Summary of the immunofluorescence seen in immunobullous disorders

| Disorder | Direct IMF | Indirect IMF |
| --- | --- | --- |
| Pemphigus vulgaris | 100% have IgG in the epidermis +/– C3 (IgA in IgA pemphigus) | Anti-epidermal IgG |
| Bullous pemphigoid | Linear IgG and/or C3 along BMZ | 70% have anti-BMZ IgG |
| Cicatricial pemphigoid | 90% linear IgG and/or C3 along BMZ (more likely on mucosal biopsy) | 20% have anti-BMZ IgG |
| Epidermolysis bullosa acquisita | Linear IgG and/or C3 along BMZ | 50% have anti-BMZ IgG |

| Gestational pemphigoid | Linear C3 BMZ +/– IgG | 100% complement added anti-BMZ IgG |
| Linear IgA disease | Linear IgA BMZ (lamina lucida) | 70% have anti-BMZ IgA |
| Dermatitis herpetiformis | Granular IgA BMZ (dermal papillae) | – |

Placing a skin biopsy in saline the epidermis and dermis split along the basement membrane zone, this salt-split sample can then be subjected to direct IMF which can give further diagnostic information.

**Table 5.12** Salt-split immunofluorescence of immunobullous disorders

| Salt-split direct IMF findings | Associations |
| --- | --- |
| Salt-split with antibodies on the roof/epidermal side | Bullous and gestational pemphigoid |
| Salt-split with antibodies on either or both sides | Cicatricial pemphigoid |
| Salt-split with antibodies on the base/dermal side | Epidermis bullosa acquisita |

In this question the patient has bullous pemphigoid, this would show IgG and/or C3 in a linear pattern along the basement membrane zone. If the sample was salt-split the antibodies would be seen on the roof/epidermal side of the biopsy. Indirect IMF of the serum would show IgG anti-basement membrane zone antibodies in 70% of patients.

## 95 D. BP antigen 2 (BP 180)
This patient has a typical presentation of gestational pemphigoid with an expected autoantibody pattern on direct IMF. In this question the target for antibodies in gestational pemphigoid is the BP antigen 2 (BP 180).

**Table 5.13** Target antigens in immunobullous disorders

| Immunobullous disorder | Target antigens |
| --- | --- |
| Pemphigus | Desmogleins 1 and 3, desmoplakins, plectin |
| Bullous pemphigoid | BP antigen 1 (BP 230), BP antigen 2 (BP 180) |
| Gestational pemphigoid | BP antigen 2 (BP 180) |
| Linear IgA disease | BP antigen 2 (BP 180), 97 kda |
| Epidermolysis bullosa acquisita | Type VII dermal collagen |

## 96 B. IgA around superficial and deep vessels

In this question a young boy is presenting with a vasculitic rash and history consistent with Henoch-Schönlein purpura. Although a number of autoantibodies may be seen on direct IMF the presence of significant amounts of IgA is typical.

**Table 5.14** Direct immunofluorescence patterns seen in non-bullous disorders

| Disorder | Direct IMF pattern |
|----------|-------------------|
| Erythema Multiforme | Superficial vessel IgG, IgM, C3, fibrinogen |
| Leukocytoclastic vasculitis | Superficial and deep vessel IgG, IgM, C3, fibrinogen |
| Henoch-Schönlein purpura | Superficial and deep vessel IgA, C3, fibrinogen |
| Livedo vasculitis | Superficial vessel wall IgM, C3 |
| Rheumatoid vasculitis | Superficial and deep vessel wall IgM, C3 |
| Porphyrias | BMZ and vessel wall IgG |
| Lupus | Stippled IgG or IgM on BMZ |

# Chapter 6

# Infectious diseases

## QUESTIONS

**97** A 47-year-old man presents with a rash on his leg. He has recently been walking in the forests of southern England and received a number of tick bites. One of these bites developed into an expanding erythematous plaque with central clearing. On examination he also has some localised lymphadenopathy in the ipsilateral groin. If this rash was not treated and the disease progressed which of the following clinical signs would you not expect to see:

A  disseminated erythema migrans
B  heart block
C  mouth ulceration
D  generalised lymphadenopathy
E  chronic arthritis.

**98** A 19-year-old man presents with a widespread rash. He has recently moved to the city to start studying at university. On examination he has a generalised papulosquamous eruption consisting of 1–20 mm sized pink-brown lesions with a collarette of scale. Of note the rash is present on his palms and soles. You suspect a diagnosis of syphilis and serology confirms your suspicion. If the patient refuses treatment a number of possible outcomes may occur with the exception of:

A  recurrence of secondary syphilis
B  re-infection with primary syphilis
C  latent syphilis with potential of reactivation
D  clearance of the disease
E  tertiary syphilis.

**99** You are asked to review a teenager from Southern Africa with eczema. During your examination you note a marked forward convexity of the right tibia and suspect this may be a sabre tibia. You request a VDRL that is positive. What is the most likely underlying diagnosis:

A   secondary syphilis
B   tertiary yaws
C   primary yaws
D   latent syphilis
E   secondary yaws.

**100** A 46-year-old man from South America presents with penile ulceration. He also has inguinal lymphadenopathy and back pain. You suspect that he may have lymphogranuloma venereum. What is the organism responsible for this condition:

A   chlamydia trachomatis
B   haemophilus ducreyi
C   calymmatobacterium (Klebsiella) granulomatis
D   herpes simplex virus
E   neisseria gonorrhoea.

**101** A patient is referred from the maxillofacial surgeons. He presented 6 months earlier with a large abscess in his mouth that spread to involve the mandible. The area has been surgically debrided and samples have grown acintomycosis species. What treatment would you recommend:

A   penicillin
B   fluconazole
C   itraconazole
D   ivermectin
E   ganciclovir.

**102** A patient presents with maceration between the toeweb spaces. There has been little response to a succession of topical imazole creams prescribed by his family doctor. When examining the area under Wood's light there is some pink fluorescence. What is the likely responsible organism:

A   erysipelothrix rhusiopathiae
B   tinea rubrum
C   trichophyton tonsurans
D   streptococcus
E   corynebacterium minutissimum.

**103** A seven-year-old girl presents with alopecia of the scalp associated with erythema, scaling and pustules. Tinea capitis is suspected and a hair pull grows trichophyton tonsurans on mycology. If treatment with griseofulvin was started what dose would you recommend for this 20 kg girl:

A   100 mg twice daily for 4 weeks
B   200 mg once daily for 6 weeks
C   400 mg once daily for 8 weeks
D   400 mg twice daily for 6 weeks
E   400 mg once daily for 12 weeks.

**104** A 32-year-old man presents after recently returning from a beach holiday. He complains that whilst he has obtained a good tan there are numerous white areas on his chest and back. On examination he has numerous small patches of hypopigmentation with overlying scale. Under Wood's light the patches fluoresce yellow. What treatment would you recommend.

A   oral griseofulvin
B   topical griseofulvin
C   oral terbinafine
D   topical terbinafine
E   topical ketoconazole.

**105** A 17-year-old man presents with maceration between the toeweb spaces of his left foot. There is also some scale on the surrounding area of the plantar foot. Skin mycology confirms your suspicion of tinea pedis. Which of the following is the most likely causative organism:

A   tinea verrucosum
B   tinea mentagrophytes
C   blastomyces dermatitidis
D   sporothrix schenckii
E   penicillium marneffei.

**106** A 73-year-old lady presents with a candidal rash beneath her breasts and in her flexural regions. Which of the following is not a risk factor for candidal infection:

A  diabetes
B  occlusion
C  hypohidrosis
D  antibiotic use
E  Cushing's syndrome.

**107** You are asked to review an unwell eight-year-old girl who is currently undergoing chemotherapy for acute lymphoblastic leukaemia. On examination she has a widespread rash consisting of vesicles on an erythematous base. Over her right buttock and extending down the leg the rash has a zosteriform appearance. You perform a Tzanck smear that shows a number of multinucleated giant cells. What treatment should you recommend:

A  send home with topical aciclovir
B  send home with oral aciclovir
C  admit to the oncology ward for IV aciclovir
D  admit to the oncology ward for oral aciclovir
E  admit to an isolation room for IV acyclovir.

**108** Herpes simplex is a:

A  double stranded DNA virus
B  single stranded DNA virus
C  double stranded RNA virus
D  single stranded RNA virus
E  mycobacterium.

**109** A 15-year-old girl presents with a diffuse maculopapular rash. She has been generally unwell for a few weeks and her general practitioner has recently given her a course of ampicillin. You suspect that she had suffered a hypersensitivity skin reaction to ampicillin due to infectious mononucleosis. The Epstein-Barr virus (EBV) is implicated in infectious mononucleosis and all of the following disorders, except:

A   erythema multiforme
B   erythema nodosum
C   oral hairy leukoplakia
D   cutaneous lichen planus
E   nasopharyngeal carcinoma.

**110** You are asked to review a three-year-old child who has been admitted under the paediatric team with a rash and systemic upset. Before seeing the patient you are taken aside by the nurse who explains that the mother is adversarial towards medical professionals and she is strong believer in 'natural' products. On examination the patient has a widespread erythematous maculopapular rash. The mother says this started on the head and spread downwards to cover much of the body. On examination of the mouth there are some grey-white papules on the oral mucosa. If this condition was to worsen which of these complications may occur:

A   encephalomyelitis
B   heart block
C   widespread venous thrombosis
D   iritis
E   haemolytic anaemia.

**111** You review a six-year-old girl known to the department with atopic eczema. She has developed a number of small, pearly umbilicated papules suggestive of molluscum contagiosum. What virus is responsible for this condition:

A   a DNA human papilloma virus
B   an RNA human papilloma virus
C   an enterovirus
D   an RNA pox virus
E   a DNA pox virus.

**112** A middle-aged patient presents who has recently emigrated from rural Mexico. On examination he has multiple nodules with ulceration and sinus tracts around the jaw line. His English is limited though he is able to convey that he has tuberculosis. What condition is he likely to have:

A   tuberculosis chancre
B   scrofuloderma
C   lupus vulgaris
D   lupus pernio
E   tuberculosis verrucosa cutis.

**113** You are asked to see a man with an inflamed nodule on the dorsum of his hand. The patient keeps a number of tropical fish as pets and you suspect infection with mycobacterium marinum. An incisional biopsy is performed which shows a granulomatous infiltrate suspicious of mycobacterial infection. What treatment would you recommend:

A   surgical excision with narrow margins
B   surgical excision with 1 cm wide margin
C   prolonged course of minocycline
D   prolonged course of isoniazid
E   short course of flucloxacillin.

**114** The lepromin skin test is strongly positive in:

A   tuberculoid leprosy
B   lepromatous leprosy
C   dimorphous leprosy
D   a type 1 reactional state in leprosy
E   a type 2 reactional state in leprosy.

**115** You are asked to review a four-year-old girl with an acute infection of her fingers. On examination the index and middle finger of the right hand are swollen with thick intact blisters and surrounding erythema. The fingers are warm and the edge of the blisters is purulent. What is the most likely organism responsible for this infection:

A   staphylococcus epidermidis
B   Klebsiella
C   staphylococcus aureas
D   mycobacterium marinum
E   group A beta-haemolytic streptococcus.

**116** A 37-year-old serviceman with the air force presents with an ulcer on his nose. He has recently returned from the Middle East and a local doctor has diagnosed the lesion as cutaneous leishmaniasis. Which of the following organisms is most likely to have infected this patient:

A   L. braziliensis
B   L. aethiopica
C   L. tropica
D   L. chagasi
E   L. donovani.

**117** A 73-year-old man returns from a trip abroad and complains of an itchy rash. Over the next few weeks his children and grandchildren also develop a similar itchy rash. On examining the patient you suspect scabies infestation and recommend the whole family is treated with malathion. Which of the following areas would you not expect to see the rash on this patient:

A   wrists
B   extensor aspect of elbows
C   face
D   genitalia
E   axillae.

**118** Which of the following statements about body louse (pediculus humanus) infestation is true:

A   The body louse is too small to see
B   The body louse feeds on shed stratum corneum
C   The body louse lives on the human skin
D   The body louse lives on clothing
E   The female louse lays up to 3000 eggs in their lifetime.

## ANSWERS

### 97 C. Mouth ulceration

This patient is presenting with a rash typical of erythema chronicum migrans, a feature of early Lyme disease. Infection is due to the gram negative spirochete Borrelia Burgdorferi, a vector-borne disease spread by ticks of the ixodes species. In Northern Europe and America the ticks are commonly found on deer and mice. The features of Lyme disease may be divided into early localised, early disseminated and chronic:

- early localised – erythema chronicum migrans, fever, localised lymphadenopathy
- early disseminated – disseminated erythema chronicum migrans, borrelial lymphocytoma, meningitis, cranial nerve palsies, acute arthritis, myositis, pericarditis, heart block and arrhythmias, generalised lymphadenopathy, conjunctivitis, iritis, hepatitis, glomerulonephritis
- chronic – acrodermatitis chronica atrophicans, encephalopathy, neuropathies, chronic arthritis.

**Table 6.1** Cutaneous features of Lyme disease

| Name | Clinical features |
| --- | --- |
| Erythema chronicum migrans | An erythematous expanding annular plaque with a light centre, the eventual diameter is variable but is often around 5 cm, the rash favours the trunk and groin and is often associated with a flu-like illness and pyrexia, it resolves over 4–6 weeks |
| Disseminated erythema chronicum migrans | Occurring a few weeks after the initial rash, a disseminated erythema migrans may occur with multiple small annular plaques |
| Borrelial lymphocytoma | Firm red-blue plaques which are seen on the earlobes and nipples often associated with lymphadenopathy, histology shows reactive lymphoid hyperplasia |
| Acrodermatitis chronica atrophicans | A chronic cutaneous feature that may occur between 6 months and 10 years following initial infection. An initial inflammatory stage with erythematous violaceous plaques and nodules is seen on the extremities. This is followed by a chronic atrophic stage with glistening appearance, prominent blood vessels, fibrous nodules, pigmentary and sensory change |

Treatment of Lyme disease is with amoxicillin or tetracyclines. In this question all the answers are possible complications of Lyme disease with the exception of mouth ulceration.

### 98 B. Re-infection with primary syphilis

This patient is presenting with a rash typical of secondary syphilis. Without treatment after 1–3 months the rash and other signs will resolve and the patient will develop latent syphilis. Latent syphilis may flare again as secondary syphilis, develop into chronic tertiary syphilis or the spirochete may be cleared and the patient cured. In this question if the patient is re-exposed to syphilis he will not develop primary disease as he either already has the disease or has developed an immune response when he cleared it.

Primary syphilis occurs 1–3 months following inoculation as a single, painless indolent ulcer on the genitalia (chancre) with regional lymphadenopathy. The ulcer heals after a few weeks and may be totally asymptomatic especially in females.

Secondary syphilis occurs 1–3 months after the primary disease as the spirochete spreads systemically through the blood and lymphoreticular system. Patients are generally unwell with a pyrexia, lethargy, sore throat, weight loss and generalised lymphadenopathy. Eighty per cent develop a pink-brown papulosquamous rash involving the palms and soles with a collarette of scale. Small mucosal ulcers may develop into large grey (snail track) plaques. Patchy alopecia may also develop. In moist creased areas broad flat wart-like growths may occur (condyloma latum). After 3–12 weeks the rash and lesions resolve into latent syphilis.

Tertiary syphilis occurs between 2 and 20 years following initial infection. Significant neurological problems may develop (neurosyphilis) as may potentially fatal involvement of the great vessels. Syphilitic tumours (gummas) may infiltrate the bones, liver and skin.

Syphilis serology is positive from two weeks after the chancre appears. The Venereal Disease Research Laboratory (VDRL) test is sensitive for active syphilis but is non-specific. A number of auto-immune disorders register a false positive VDRL. There are other more specific tests such as the fluorescent treponemal antibody-absorption (FTA), this is less helpful as it remains positive when the syphilis has been cleared. Treatment is with penicillin.

## 99 B. Tertiary yaws

Sabre tibia is a marked forward convexity of the tibia due to gumma formation and periostitis in either tertiary syphilis or tertiary yaws. Yaws is a tropical infection due to the spirochete treponema pallidum pertenue which is closely related to the syphilic spirochete treponema pallidum pallidum. Yaws is found in the tropical regions of South America, Asia, Africa and South-East Asia. It is transmitted by skin-to-skin contact between an infective lesion and a defect in the epidermal surface such as an abrasion. Once infected a three stage process occurs similar to syphilis.

Primary yaws (Mother yaws). At the site of inoculation a red painless infiltrated papule occurs, this enlarges up to 5 cm then breaks down into an ulcer with a yellow crust. It occurs from 10 days after infection and heals over 3–6 months. Plantar hyperkeratosis may also be seen in this stage.

Secondary yaws (Daughter yaws). Months to years later multiple widespread skin lesions occur often adjacent to orifices (nose, mouth). These again may break down into ulcers and take up to six months to heal.

Tertiary yaws. Ten per cent of people develop tertiary disease which occurs 5–10 years following initial infection. Abscesses occur that necrose and ulcerate forming tracts, sinuses, scarring and deformity. Destruction is seen in the bones, joints and soft tissues. Typical features include the sabre tibia and rhinopharyngitis mutilans.

Diagnosis may be by dark field microscopy of samples from early lesions or serology which is indistinguishable from syphilis. Treatment is with antibiotics such as penicillin. In this question the most likely diagnosis is tertiary yaws as the patient has emigrated from an endemic area.

## 100 A. Chlamydia trachomatis

There are a number of causes of penile ulceration:
- inflammatory – Reiter's syndrome, lupus, Behçet's syndrome, pemphigus, Stevens-Johnson syndrome, erosive balanitis
- infective – chancroid, syphilis, HSV, granuloma inguinale, lymphogranuloma venereum, candida
- other – trauma, neoplasms.

Lymphogranuloma venereum is a rare sexually transmitted disease more commonly seen in tropical countries and homosexual individuals. In answer to the question it is caused by the organism chlamydia trachomatis. Primary disease is seen 3–12 days following inoculation as a penile papule, erosion, ulcer or vesicle. This is associated with a non-specific urethritis and regional lymphadenopathy. Left untreated it may progress to an inguinal syndrome with inguinal lymphadenopathy, fever and back pain. The inguinal lymph nodes may rupture leading to sinuses and fistulae. Ano-genital-rectal syndrome may also be seen with proctocolitis, rectal abscesses and fistulae. The organism may be identified by PCR and treated with erythromycin or doxycycline.

Haemophilus ducreyi is responsible for chancroid, a sexually transmitted disease seen in developing countries. Acute, painful genital ulcers occur alongside regional lymphadenopathy. It does not produce systemic disease and may be treated with tetracyclines or sulphonamide antibiotics. Calymmatobacterium (Klebsiella) granulomatis is responsible for granuloma inguinale (donovanosis) a rare, chronic, ulcerative bacterial infection seen in developing countries. A classical painless 'beefy' red ulcer is seen. Treatment is with doxycycline.

## 101 A. Penicillin
Acintomycosis is a rare anaerobic bacterial infection that causes painful abscesses in the mouth, neck, lungs and gastrointestinal tract. The abscesses grow slowly over many months invading bone, muscle and soft tissues. Sinuses may form to the skin producing a purulent discharge with 'sulphur' granules. There are often predisposing factors, for example recent dental work or immunodeficiency. The answer to this question is treatment with antibiotics such as penicillin, not antifungals or antivirals.

## 102 E. Corynebacterium minutissimum
In this question the patient is presenting with erythrasma, a superficial mild skin infection due to the gram positive bacteria corynebacterium minutissimum. Commoner in people with diabetes, patients present with pink-red well defined patches in moist flexural areas. There is an overlying fine scale and with time the colour changes from pink-red to brown. Under Wood's light erythrasma fluoresces 'coral' pink. Treatment is with antibiotics such as erythromycin.

Corynebacterium minutissimum also causes trichomycosis axillaris a superficial infection of axillary and pubic hair. Patients present with adherent yellow-red-black nodular cylinders attached to the hair shafts. Treatment is shaving, antibacterial soaps and antibiotics. Corynebacterium is also a cause of pitted keratolysis alongside actinomyces and micrococcus sedentarius.

Erysipelothrix rhusiopathiae is a bacteria which can affect the skin causing red-purple plaques (erysipeloid) and rarely disseminates where it may cause subacute bacterial endocarditis. It is an occupational infection picked up from shellfish, birds and mammals. Treatment is with penicillins or cephalosporins.

## 103 C. 400 mg once daily for 8 weeks

Tinea capitis is a superficial fungal infection of the scalp and hair. It is most common in prepubescent children. After puberty the composition of sebum changes and it becomes more anti-fungal. Infection occurs through airborne spread or contact and there is a significant reservoir of potentially infectious asymptomatic carriers in the population. Once infected, the patient develops itching and hair loss associated with scaling, erythema, pustules and broken hair stubs. On occasions a highly inflamed kerion may form with bogginess, pustules and overlying crust. The fungal organisms may originate from other humans (microsporum audouinii, trichophyton tonsurans), animals (microsporum canis) or rarely soil (microsporum gypseum). Microsporum canis infection fluoresces green under Wood's light, other infections do not. Treatment is with antifungals such as griseofulvin, terbinafine and itraconazole. The normal dose for griseofulvin is 10 mg/kg for 6–8 weeks. In this question the patient has trichophyton tonsurans which requires a higher dose of 20 mg/kg for 6–8 weeks.

## 104 E. Topical ketoconazole

This patient has tinea versicolor a superficial infection with the yeast malassezia furfur (pityrosporum orbiculare). It is a common infection in young adults that may become widespread in patients with diabetes and Cushing's disease. There is an asymptomatic, asymmetrical rash of hypo or hyperpigmentation with overlying scale that fluoresces yellow under Wood's light. As the infection is a yeast it does not respond to griseofulvin or terbinafine. Treatment is with selenium sulphide or an imazole antifungal. In this question topical ketoconazole would be appropriate.

## 105 B. Tinea mentagrophytes

Tinea pedis is a superficial fungal infection of the foot and toeweb spaces. It is commonly due to the organism tinea rubrum and in this question tinea mentagrophytes. Tinea verrucosum is a zoophilic organism often responsible for Tinea barbae, fungal infection of the beard area. Tinea barbae may present severely with multiple pustules, abscesses, tracts, alopecia, kerion, systemic upset and localised lymphadenopathy.

Tinea unguium (onychomycosis) is fungal infection of the nails, it is much more common in toe nails than finger nails and is strongly associated with tinea pedis. It is often due to T. rubrum, T. mentagrophytes and epidermophyton floccosum, but may also be due to yeasts and moulds such as aspergillus. Treatment is with prolonged courses of systemic antifungals such as terbinafine. Both tinea unguium and tinea pedis are strong risk factors for acute lower limb bacterial cellulitis.

Tinea corporis is a superficial fungal infection of the trunk and limbs. It is more common in tropical countries and strongly associated with tinea pedis and tinea capitis. Risk factors include communal living, wrestling, gym usage and immunosuppression. It is often due to the organisms T. rubrum and T. mentagrophytes. Tinea incognito occurs when tinea corporis is mistakenly treated with a topical steroid. It may be difficult to diagnose due to the lack of scale. Majocchi's granuloma is a rare complication which occurs in ladies with tinea pedis who shave their legs. Follicular infection with T. rubrum results, which may be extensive.

Tinea cruris is a superficial fungal infection of the inguinal region and inner thighs; it may spread to the abdomen and buttocks. It is more common in obese males and hot countries. A sharply demarcated, scaly advancing border distinguishes it from flexural psoriasis. Tinea manuum is a superficial fungal infection of the palms. It presents with unilateral, non-inflamed hyperkeratosis and scaling. Both tinea cruris and tinea manuum are often due to the organisms T. rubrum, T. mentagrophytes and epidermophyton floccosum.

Blastomyces dermatitidis, sporothrix schenckii and penicillium marneffei are opportunistic fungi responsible for the infections blastomycosis, sporotrichosis and penicilliosis respectively.

## 106 C. Hypohidrosis

Risk factors for candidal infection include:

- diabetes
- occlusion
- hyperhidrosis
- steroids
- Cushing's syndrome
- antibiotics
- immunosuppression
- hypothyroidism
- hypoparathyroidism
- xerostomia (oral candida).

Candia is a commensal saprophyte which does not fluoresce with Wood's light, common species include candida albicans and candida tropicalis. Candida infection may present anywhere on the skin or mucous membranes with a number of patterns.

**Table 6.2** Cutaneous manifestations of candida infection

| Name | Clinical features |
| --- | --- |
| Oral candida | Denture stomatitis, angular cheilitis, thrush (white exudates), chronic atrophic (patchy erythema), chronic hyperplastic (adherent white plaques), glossitis (painful atrophy of tongue) |
| Genital candida | Vulvovaginitis, balanitis, superimposed infection on napkin dermatitis |
| Skin candida | Candidal intertrigo, erythematous or erosive patches with satellite pustules |
| Nail candida | Periungual candidiasis, nail plate infection |
| Systemic candida | Seen in immunocompromised, poor prognosis, includes candidal endocarditis |

Chronic mucocutaneous candidiasis is a manifestation of a number of primary immunodeficiencies. Patients present with chronic, treatment resistant infections of the nails, skin and mucosa which may be granulomatous. Some patients have associated endocrinopathies, vitiligo and alopecia.

In this question hypohidrosis is not a risk factor for candidal infection, although hyperhidrosis is.

**107 E. Admit to an isolation room for IV aciclovir**
In this question a young girl is presenting with disseminated **zoster** (shingles). She has been previously infected with the herpes zoster virus (HZV) and would have presented with varicella (chickenpox) at that

time. Subsequently her chemotherapy has led to immunosuppression and reactivation of HZV in a disseminated pattern. The patient is systemically unwell; she needs an intravenous anti-viral medication such as aciclovir. She has intact vesicles and is therefore infectious so should not be admitted to the oncology ward where she might infect other immunosuppressed patients. The patient should also avoid pregnant women and babies.

Varicella (chickenpox) is commonly seen in children as a manifestation of primary HZV infection. After an incubation of 10–23 days patients present with an eruption of pruritic erythematous nodules and macules starting on the scalp and trunk and spreading outwards. Over 12–24 hours distinct 1–3 mm clear vesicles form with a surrounding red halo, there may be only a few vesicles or many hundreds. With time the vesicles become pustular then crust over. New crops of vesicles occur allowing lesions at all stages to be seen on the same patient. The patient is highly contagious from four days prior to the rash appearing until all the lesions have crusted over. Infection is by droplet spread and transplacentally which may lead to significant teratogenicity. Complications include myocarditis, meningitis, pneumonia, hepatitis and arthritis.

Zoster (shingles) occurs due to reactivation of HZV infection with illness, age, malignancy, steroids or immunosuppression. Reactivation occurs from the sensory and motor root ganglions leading to a unilateral dermatomal pattern of painful pruritic vesicles that last 2–3 weeks. Five per cent of patients may develop recurrent shingles occurring along the same dermatome. Disseminated zoster may occur in immunosuppressed patients with greater than 20 vesicles present outside of the dermatome. These patients are at risk of systemic complications such as meningitis. Patients with active zoster are infectious to those who have not had varicella and should avoid non-immune pregnant women and babies. Up to 10–15% of patients with zoster develop a post-herpetic neuralgia which may resolve with time or become chronic. If trigeminal nerve involvement is suspected the patient should be urgently referred to an ophthalmologist due to the risk of ocular keratitis.

## 108 A. Double stranded DNA virus
All the viruses in the herpes family have a double stranded DNA structure including herpes simplex virus (HSV). Like in HZV a Tzanck smear from the base of freshly burst vesicles shows multinucleate giant cells.

HSV is transmitted by direct contact and has a 3–14 day incubation period. Primary infection may be severe with extensive vesicles and pustular lesions or be totally asymptomatic. Complications include herpetic stomatitis, keratoconjunctivitis, encephalitis, pharyngitis, meningitis and vulvovaginitis. Following acute infection the virus lays dormant in sensory root ganglion and may be reactivated as recurrent secondary disease. This often presents as recurrent cold sores (HSV1) or recurrent genital herpes (HSV2). HSV infection can be associated with recurrent erythema multiforme and can infect eczema causing Kaposi's varicelliform eruption (eczema herpeticum).

**Table 6.3** Members of the human herpes virus family

| Human herpes type | Name | Clinical features |
| --- | --- | --- |
| 1 | Herpes simplex 1 (HSV-1) | Cold sores, keratitis |
| 2 | Herpes simplex 2 (HSV-2) | Genital herpes |
| 3 | Herpes zoster virus (HZV) | Varicella, zoster |
| 4 | Epstein-Barr virus (EBV) | Infectious mononucleosis, lymphomas |
| 5 | Cytomegalovirus (CMV) | TORCH, CMV retinitis |
| 6 | Herpes lymphotropic virus | Roseola |
| 7 | Human herpes virus 7 | Roseola |
| 8 | Human herpes virus 8 | Kaposi's sarcoma |

## 109 D. Cutaneous lichen planus

Although the Epstein-Barr virus (EBV) has been associated with oral lichen planus (LP), no association exists with cutaneous LP. Most EBV infections occur in childhood and result in a subclinical or mild non-specific illness. If EBV infection occurs later patients may develop infectious mononucleosis (glandular fever). Transmission is by saliva where the virus targets and infects B-cells.

Infectious mononucleosis presents in teenagers after a 1–2 month incubation with pharyngitis, fever and lymphadenopathy. Other features may include headache, malaise, hepatosplenomegaly, anorexia, cough, arthralgia, eyelid and buccal petechiae, periorbital oedema and a non-specific exanthem which may be morbilliform, urticarial, pustular or petechial. Complications include hepatitis, thrombocytopenia, haemolytic anaemia, glomerulonephritis and neurological disease. If ampicillin is given a hypersensitivity skin reaction may occur with a widespread maculopapular rash which may become confluent. The reaction occurs less frequently with amoxicillin, penicillin and cephalosporins. Infectious mononucleosis tends to resolve in 2–3 weeks.

A number of other conditions have been associated with EBV infection, including:
- B and T-cell lymphomas
- oral hairy leukoplakia
- nasopharyngeal carcinoma
- post-transplant lymphoproliferative disorders
- Gianotti Crosti syndrome
- erythema multiforme
- erythema nodosum
- urticaria
- erythema annulare centrifugum
- pityriasis lichenoides
- acrocyanosis
- genital ulcers
- Kikuchi's syndrome.

Cytomegalovirus (CMV) infection is subclinical in 95% of immunocompetent patients. The virus is transmitted in body fluids and has a 1–2 month incubation period. If an immunocompetent patient develops symptoms the picture is similar to infectious mononucleosis. In immunocompromised patients CMV may occur as a primary infection or be reactivated. Serious complications may occur including CMV retinitis and CMV encephalitis. Transplacental spread of CMV during pregnancy may lead to TORCH syndrome with severe congenital malformations and a 'blueberry muffin' rash. Treatment is with ganciclovir.

## 110 A. Encephalomyelitis
This three-year-old child is presenting with measles. The history is of systemic upset, a maculopapular rash with cephalocaudal spread and mouth lesions typical of Koplik's spots. The mother's attitude towards conventional medicine is an indicator that the child may not have received the MMR (measles, mumps and rubella) vaccine. Measles is a paramyxovirus which presents with a prodrome of lethargy, cough and conjunctivitis. Koplik's spots appear on the 2nd day of the illness and the rash appears on day 3 or 4 and lasts for 5 days. In answer to the

question complications include encephalomyelitis, otitis, pneumonia and myocarditis.

**Table 6.4** Common viral exanthems

| Name | Clinical features |
|------|-------------------|
| Rubella (german measles) | A mild, self-limiting exanthem of rose-pink macules with cephalocaudal spread. Oral lesions may occur, occipital lymphadenopathy is common as is arthralgia and myalgia. Infection in pregnancy may lead to severe teratogenicity |
| Roseola infantum (Sixth disease) | Infants and young children present with 2–5 days of high fever followed by a rash of small pink papules on the head and trunk. The rash lasts 1–2 days and is due to HHV6 and 7 |
| STAR complex | Sore throat, arthritis and rash, commonly due to rubella and parvovirus B19 |
| Hand, foot and mouth disease | A benign self-limiting coxsackie virus infection, patients have fever, malaise a vesicular eruption on the palms and soles and erosive stomatitis |

## 111 E. A DNA pox virus

Molluscum contagiosum is caused by a DNA pox virus called the molluscum contagiosum virus (MCV). Infection occurs in children and the immunocompromised. It is more commonly seen in atopics. Atypical and widespread lesions may be a presenting feature of HIV.

**Table 6.5** Cutaneous disorders caused by pox viruses

| Name | Clinical features |
|------|-------------------|
| Orf | A papule or nodule on the hand seen in animal workers, resolves in 1–2 months without scarring |
| Milker's nodule | Similar presentation to Orf |
| Smallpox | Now eradicated, variola major was potentially life threatening |
| Vaccina | Cowpox virus used for vaccination against smallpox, a live vaccine that may cause local infection at the site of vaccination |
| Monkeypox | Seen in Africa, patients present with centrifugal vesicopustules and lymphadenopathy |
| Cowpox | Caught from cats, similar to Orf but heals with scarring |

Viral warts are due to the human papilloma virus (HPV), a circular double stranded DNA virus which is highly specific for skin and mucosa. There are over 200 types of HPV, some of which are oncogenic.

**Table 6.6** Common patterns of viral wart infection

| Type of wart | % | Features | HPV types |
|---|---|---|---|
| Common (verrucca vulgaris) | 70% | Flesh coloured, rough, hyperkeratotic papules | 2, 4, 29 |
| Plantar palmar | 35% | Thick, hyperkeratotic lesions | 1 ,2, 4, 10 |
| Flat (verrucca plana) | 5% | Small, flat topped, multiple, may hyperpigment | 3, 10 |
| Anogenital (condyloma acuminatum) | – | Moist, cauliflower like, can be sexually transmitted, more common in homosexual men and children | 6, 11, 42–44 |

## 112 B. Scrofuloderma

In this question the patient has scrofuloderma, a cutaneous variant of tuberculosis (TB). Commonly seen around the jaw-line the infection starts from a deep subcutaneous nodule (cold abscess) and drains to the skin with ulceration and sinus tracts. Multiple blue heaped up ulcers are characteristic. Lupus pernio is a cutaneous variant of sarcoidosis not tuberculosis. Other forms of cutaneous TB include the following.

Tuberculosis chancre – direct inoculation of TB into the skin causes a painless, firm enlarging papulo-nodule after 2–4 weeks. The nodule may enlarge and ulcerate causing localised lymphadenopathy. Eventually it either heals spontaneously or may develop into another form of cutaneous TB.

Tuberculosis verrucosa cutis – inoculation of the skin by TB at a site prone to trauma leads to a small indurated wart-like papule. With time this develops into a red-brown verrucous plaque and may have a central abscess.

Oro-facial TB – autoinoculation of TB to the mucosa or skin adjacent to orifices infected with TB. Most commonly seen in or around the mouth in patients with pulmonary TB. A red plaque is seen that ulcerates and tends to resolve spontaneously.

Lupus vulgaris – cutaneous TB infection in a patient with a strong immune response leads to lupus vulgaris. Red-brown plaques are seen with 'apple-jelly' papulo-nodules. It heals with scarring. Most often seen on the head and neck the lesions may be ulcerative, vegetating or tumour like.

Miliary TB – systemic, septic spread of TB leading to multiple widespread pin-head sized blue-red papulo-vesicles that heal with scarring. The lesions may grow into a subcutaneous nodule that ulcerates and forms a sinus tract, a TB gumma.

Tuberculids – a descriptive term for a number of rashes that have been associated with systemic TB infection. Includes erythema induratum (Bazin's disease), nodular vasculitis, erythema nodosum, lichen scrofulosorum and papulonecrotic tuberculid.

## 113 C. Prolonged course of minocycline

Mycobacterium marinum is a disease of fish and water, there needs to be a portal of entry such as a graze for infection to occur in humans. When infection occurs it presents as a blue-red inflammatory nodule (a fish tank granuloma) often on the hand or arm which may ulcerate and form an abscess. Multiple lesions may occur following the path of lymphatic drainage and in the immunocompromised the infection may become disseminated. In answer to the question treatment is with antibiotics such as tetracyclines. There is often resistance to isoniazid.

Other atypical mycobacterial skin infections include the following.

Mycobacterium ulcerans (Buruli ulcer, bairnsdale ulcer, searles ulcer) – causes indolent ulceration which can be giant (↑15 cm), more common in tropical countries and children. The infection starts as a nodule which breaks down into a painless, deep necrotic ulcer often on the legs. Surgery is the treatment of choice, antimicrobial medications are not effective.

Mycobacterium Kansasii – similar to TB, it is often seen in middle-aged, white, affluent men of Northern Europe. Most often presenting as a lung infection it can cause skin nodules, plaques and ulcers. If immunocompromised the infection may become disseminated. Treatment is with anti-TB medications.

M. fortuitum, M. chelonae, M. abscessus – organisms are found in water and soil; infection presents as multiple erythematous nodules on a limb that may ulcerate and cause cellulitis, abscess or sinus. Treatment is with antibiotics.

M. avium, M. intracellulare – two similar mycobacterium. They most often cause lung infection in immunocompromised patients. Rarely they may also infect the skin causing an ulcer or papulopustules.

M. scrofulaceum – similar to M. avium but is a benign, self-limiting disease. Patients present with cervical lymphadenopathy and sinus formation indistinguishable from scrofuloderma. Treatment is surgical.

## 114 A. Tuberculoid leprosy

The lepromin skin test is used to determine the patient's immune response to leprosy. Killed bacillus is injected intradermally. In answer to the question if a strong type IV reaction occurs this is suggestive of tuberculoid leprosy, a weak or negative reaction suggests lepromatous leprosy.

Leprosy is a chronic, granulomatous disorder due to infection with mycobacterium leprae. It is most commonly seen in children and young adults and is endemic in a number of countries such as India and Brazil. Primary infection with leprosy causes an erythematous or hypopigmented macule and is referred to as indeterminate leprosy. The infection may fully resolve or it may also progress into any of the three main types of leprosy depending on the host's immune response. If there is a strong immune response tuberculoid leprosy will occur. If the immune response is poor it will lead to lepromatous leprosy and an intermediate response will lead to dimorphous leprosy. Dimorphous or borderline leprosy is unstable and can undergo a type 1 reactional state as it evolves into tuberculoid disease.

Table 6.7 Key features of tuberculoid and lepromatous leprosy

| Tuberculoid | Lepromatous (90% cases) |
| --- | --- |
| High degree of immunity to M. leprae | Low degree of immunity to M. leprae |
| Few skin lesions and few active organisms | Many skin lesions and millions of active organisms |
| 2–5 year incubation | 8–12 year incubation |
| Small number of large, asymmetrical, anaesthetic, hypopigmented, rough, scaly, sharp edged skin lesions; hypotrichosis and sweating | Numerous small, symmetrical, smooth skin lesions with vague edge and variable sensation; hyperpigmented papules and nodules; palpable nerves, flat nasal bridge, neuropathy, atrophy of the small muscles of hand; areas of cutaneous anaesthesia, nasal stuffiness, eye infection, loss of eyebrows; peripheral patchy neuropathy worse in cooler areas, neuropathic ulcers; loose teeth; leonine facies; testicular atrophy, impotence and gynaecomastia |

Leprosy may be diagnosed on key clinical features such as cutaneous anaesthesia and peripheral nerve enlargement. Biopsies may

117

also be taken from the raised margin of skin lesions with bacillus being shown with a fite stain. A slit skin smear may also be taken. Treatment of leprosy is with dapsone, rifampicin, clofazimine and ethionamide.

### 115 E. Group A beta-haemolytic streptococcus

In this question a young patient is presenting with the rare disorder blistering distal dactylitis. This disorder of young children present with tender bullae on an erythematous base frequently on the volar fat pads of the fingers. It is most commonly due to group A beta-haemolytic streptococcus, but has also been seen with staphylococcus aureas.

Impetigo is a common superficial bacterial infection of the skin. It is often seen on the face of children presenting with honey coloured crusts overlying superficial erosions. Initial infection is often due to streptococcus with later secondary staphylococcal involvement. Staphylococcal impetigo may present with thin flaccid blisters due to splitting of the stratum corneum by exfoliative toxins A and B. Ecthyma is a severe streptococcal impetigo with thick crust overlying punched out ulceration of the epidermis that may heal with scarring.

Erysipelas is due to superficial infection of the subcutaneous tissues. Some authors do not distinguish it from cellulitis which is considered to be a deeper infection. Most often due to streptococci patients present with a well defined, warm, erythematous plaque and systemic upset.

Furuncles and carbuncles are due to infections of hair follicles with staphylococcus that form boils and abscesses.

Staphylococcal scalded skin syndrome (SSSS) is seen in neonates and infants who cannot excrete staphylococcal exotoxins. Patients start with a rash similar to bullous impetigo and this rapidly develops into flaccid bullae and tender erythema with an oozing base. The children are unwell with fever and there is an associated mortality often due to fluid and electrolyte imbalance.

Toxic shock syndrome occurs when staphylococcal exotoxins are released into the blood stream leading to hypotension, pharyngeal oedema, conjunctival injection, diffuse erythema and desquamatization of the palms and soles. Common sites of infection include tampons, abscesses and wound infections.

## 116 C. L. tropica

Leishmaniasis is caused by protozoa of the genus leishmania, it is found throughout the world and is most commonly seen in the Middle East, South Asia and South America. Sand flies of the family phlebotominae are the vector for the disease. The clinical picture of infection depends on the species of leishmania and may vary from a self-limiting skin infection through to a fatal visceral disease. In this question the patient has developed cutaneous leishmaniasis whilst in the Middle East, the most likely responsible species is L. tropica.

**Table 6.8** Species of leishmania and their clinical picture

| Species | Clinical picture | Geographical area affected |
|---|---|---|
| L. tropica, L. Major | Cutaneous leishmaniasis | Middle East, Asia, North Africa |
| L. amazonensis | Cutaneous leishmaniasis | Central and South America |
| L. braziliensis | Cutaneous and mucocutaneous leishmaniasis | Central and South America |
| L. mexicana | Cutaneous and diffuse cutaneous leishmaniasis | Central and South America |
| L. aethiopica | Cutaneous, mucocutaneous and diffuse cutaneous leishmaniasis | North Africa |
| L. infantum | Cutaneous and visceral leishmaniasis | North Africa |
| L. chagasi | Visceral leishmaniasis | Central and South America |
| L. donovani | Visceral leishmaniasis | India, Africa |

Cutaneous leishmaniasis presents as a small red papule that darkens and breaks down into an ulcer with raised edges, it is most commonly seen on the face and extremities.

Mucocutaneous leishmaniasis occurs as sores in the nose and mouth and may also involve the skin. Untreated the mucosal lesions cause erosion and deformity of the palate, nasal septum and lips. The lesions are painful and may become secondarily infection.

Diffuse cutaneous leishmaniasis results from cutaneous disease which has spread to cover much of the skin. A chronic eruption occurs of non-ulcerative nodules which slowly progresses and is difficult to treat.

Visceral leishmaniasis (Kala azar) affects the internal organs leading to hepatosplenomegaly, anaemia, leucopoenia, fever, weakness, diarrhoea and cachexia.

Diagnosis is with skin biopsy, in most cases the protozoa can be seen on histology. Treatment is with sodium stibogluconate or meglumine antimoniate.

### 117 C. Face
Scabies infestation is caused by the mite sarcoptes scabiei var hominis. It may be caught from other humans and over 40 different animal species. The female mite burrows into the epidermis where it lays eggs. The mites themselves and their waste products cause severe pruritus. Patients present with an insidious onset of red pruritic papules and severe pruritus. With time burrows can be seen and less commonly pustules and blisters may occur. Commonly affected areas include the web-spaces between fingers, the wrists, extensor surface of the elbows, axillae, abdomen, genitals, buttocks and thighs. In answer to the question it does not tend to affect the face in adults but may do so in children. Treatment may be with malathion, permethrin, ivermectin or sulphur ointment.

Norwegian scabies is seen in the elderly or immunocompromised, there is massive infestation with mites leading to hyperplasia of the epidermis giving a 'crusted' appearance.

### 118 D. The body louse lives on clothing
The body louse (pediculus humanus var capitus) is closely related to the head louse (pediculus humanus capitis) and the pubic louse (pthirus pubis). All the insects live off human blood and thrive in unhygienic, crowded conditions. The body louse is 1–3 mm long, visible with the naked eye and lives on unwashed clothing. Female lice live for 1–3 months and lay up to 300 eggs in their lifetime. The lice are rarely seen on the skin and patients present with non-specific papules and hyperpigmentation. Treatments are similar to scabies (see above). In answer to the question the lice live on clothing not human skin.

# Chapter 7
# Lesions, surgery and skin cancer

## QUESTIONS

**119** A 63-year-old woman presents with a non-healing lesion on her right temple that has been present for over two years. On examination there is a 6 mm well defined lesion with central ulceration, telangiectasia and a shiny, rolled edge. What is the treatment of choice for this lesion:

A   superficial radiotherapy
B   single pass curettage
C   excision with 2 mm margins
D   excision with 4 mm margins
E   Mohs micrographic surgery.

**120** A 78-year-old patient is seen following excision and skin grafting of a basal cell carcinoma (BCC) from the right inner canthus. The pathology report states that the BCC was incompletely excised at the lateral peripheral margin. What would be the treatment of choice:

A   observe and treat if it recurs
B   radiotherapy to the skin graft site
C   excision of the lateral aspect of the skin graft and 4 mm additional tissue
D   Mohs micrographic surgery to the area lateral to the skin graft
E   excision of the skin graft and Mohs micrographic surgery to the whole site.

**121** You review a 53-year-old man from whom you have excised two lesions. Histology shows:

- lesion A: a well differentiated SCC arising on the scalp within an area of Bowen's disease, lesion diameter 21 mm, invading 5 mm into the deep dermis, fully excised with 2 mm histological margins; clinically 5 mm surgical margins were taken and the lesion was excised to the depth of subcutaneous fat
- lesion B: a moderately differentiated SCC arising on the scalp, lesion diameter 8 mm, invading 2 mm into upper dermis, fully excised with 3 mm histological margins; clinically 7 mm surgical margins were taken and the lesion was excised to aponeurosis.

What treatment option is most appropriate for these lesions:

A   neither lesion requires further treatment
B   lesion A requires re-excision, lesion B does not
C   lesion B requires re-excision, lesion A does not
D   both lesions require re-excision
E   both lesions require radiotherapy.

**122** An 81-year-old woman presents with a rapidly growing lesion on her right helix. On examination there is a 2 cm diameter, well defined, skin coloured nodule with a central keratin plug. You suspect a diagnosis of keratoacanthoma. What treatment option should you recommend:

A   radiotherapy
B   punch biopsy
C   incisional biopsy
D   excision biopsy
E   curettage and cautery.

**123** A 28-year-old woman presents with a history of a longstanding mole on her leg that has recently increased in size and become darker. On examination the mole stands out, it has an irregular, ill-defined border, variation in colour and it lacks symmetry. You excise the mole with 2 mm clinical margins. Histopathology reports a fully excised invasive melanoma, Breslow thickness 0.2 mm, Clark level II and no ulceration. What further treatment should you recommend:

A no further treatment is required
B re-excision of 8 mm around the scar
C re-excision of 1 cm around the scar
D re-excision of 2 cm around the scar
E refer for radiotherapy.

**124** You review a 38-year-old woman who presented two years previously with a 5.4 mm Breslow thickness melanoma on her ankle. The melanoma was removed with a 3 cm wide excision and a split skin graft was used to cover the defect. She re-presented two weeks ago with a blue-black nodule adjacent to the skin graft and palpable lymphadenopathy in the ipsilateral groin. Fine needle aspiration of the lump and groin lymph nodes has shown melanoma and a CT scan has shown no further evidence of metastatic spread. What treatment would you recommend for this patient:

A no active treatment, palliation only
B excision of the local cutaneous metastasis and radiotherapy to the groin
C excision of the local cutaneous metastasis and selective removal of enlarged lymph nodes in the groin
D excision of the local cutaneous metastasis and block lymph node dissection in the groin
E isolated limb infusion of the leg.

**125** A 34-year-old woman presents with a history of a slowly enlarging lesion on her abdomen. It started as an area of thickened skin and developed into a nodule with a blue hue. Biopsy has shown a fibrohistiocytic lesion with malignant change. What is the most likely diagnosis:

A dermatofibrosarcoma protuberans
B Merkel cell carcinoma
C angiosarcoma
D Kaposi's sarcoma
E Liposarcoma.

**126** A 77-year-old man presents with an enlarging 3 cm diameter nodule on his scalp. A diagnostic excision is performed with 2 mm peripheral margins to the level of subcutaneous fat. Histology from the lesion shows a large dermal tumour composed of fibrocystic, spindle-shaped and anaplastic cells. A number of bizarre multinucleated giant cells are seen that contain lipid. The tumour has been excised completely with a minimal margin of 0.5 mm to the deep margin. What treatment would you recommend to the patient:

A   no more treatment is required
B   re-excision with 2 cm margins
C   Mohs micrographic surgery
D   refer for radiotherapy
E   refer for chemotherapy.

**127** A 55-year-old woman presents with a rather non-descript painless nodule on her scalp. A biopsy is performed which shows adenocarcinoma. What is the most relevant investigation to perform in this patient:

A   colonoscopy
B   gastroscopy
C   mammogram
D   transvaginal ultrasound
E   MRI of the brain.

**128** A 46-year-old man presents for review after excision of a sebaceous adenoma from his chest. Of note the patient has had previous sebaceous adenomas and a sebaceous carcinoma excised. His mother has had similar problems in the past. What other specialty should you refer this patient to for further investigation:

A   cardiology
B   neurology
C   rheumatology
D   gastroenterology
E   haematology.

**129** A 26-year-old patient is referred with a number of non-pruritic plum coloured plaques on his torso; some of the plaques have central vesiculation. The patient has had recent weight loss and has been feeling non-specifically unwell. A biopsy of one of the plaques shows a dense neutrophilic infiltrate throughout the dermis. Which of the following malignancies is most likely in this patient:

A   prostate carcinoma
B   gastric adenocarcinoma
C   glucagonoma
D   clear cell carcinoma of the lung
E   acute myeloid leukaemia.

**130** Which of the following is not an appropriate treatment for early-stage mycosis fungoides:

A   topical corticosteroids
B   bexarotene
C   UVB phototherapy
D   PUVA phototherapy
E   topical nitrogen mustard.

**131** What is the commonest cause of leukaemia cutis:

A   chronic lymphocytic leukaemia
B   acute lymphocytic leukaemia
C   chronic myeloid leukaemia
D   acute myeloid leukaemia
E   monomyelocytic leukaemia.

**132** A 71-year-old lady attends your surgical list for excision of a basal cell carcinoma overlying her zygomatic arch. Whilst obtaining consent you inform her of the risk of damage to the temporal branch of the facial nerve. The patient asks what would happen if this nerve was transacted. What is the most accurate answer:

A   inability to raise the forehead on the ipsilateral side and possible ptosis
B   inability to raise the forehead on the contralateral side and possible ptosis
C   loss of sensation to the ipsilateral forehead and anterior scalp
D   loss of sensation to the contralateral forehead and anterior scalp
E   nothing – there is contralateral innervation to the forehead.

**133** What is the maximum safe dose of 1% lignocaine (lidocaine) with 1/80 000 adrenalin (epinephrine) that you can administer to a 70 kg man:

A    20 mls
B    100 mls
C    50 mls
D    10 mls
E    500 mls.

**134** An obese 44-year-old woman presents with a 'dirty' rash in her axillae. On examination she has velvety hyperpigmentation and skin tags in her axillae consistent with acanthosis nigricans. Which of the following does not have a known association with this disorder:

A    gastric adenocarcinoma
B    type 2 diabetes
C    lung carcinoma
D    minocycline treatment
E    Cushing's disease.

**135** Which of the following groups of people do not have an increased risk for developing Kaposi's sarcoma:

A    HIV positive individuals
B    homosexual males
C    elderly Africans
D    Ashkenazi Jews
E    individuals who have previously received radiotherapy treatment.

**136** Which of the following is not a recognised cause of xanthomas:

A    ritonavir
B    alcohol abuse
C    haemochromatosis
D    nephrotic syndrome
E    hyperthyroidism.

**137** A 19-year-old girl presents with a number of new lesions on her chest. The lesions are vascular with a central arteriole and radiating fine vessels. Compression of the central arteriole results in the whole lesion blanching. Which of the following may be a risk factor for developing these lesions:

A prematurity
B beta-blockers
C Mediterranean descent
D the oral contraceptive pill
E Sturge-Weber syndrome.

**138** A 52-year-old patient presents with a 9 mm basal cell carcinoma overlying the superior sternum. It is planned to remove the lesion by excision with direct closure. Which of the following medications may increase the risk of the patient developing a keloid scar:

A isotretinoin
B sumatriptan
C atenolol
D levothyroxine
E aspirin.

**139** The commonest site for chondrodermatitis nodularis helicis (CNH) in women is:

A superior helix
B tragus
C inferior helix
D antihelix
E scapha.

## ANSWERS

### 119 D. Excision with 4 mm margins

Basal cell carcinoma (BCC) is the commonest malignancy seen in humans. They are low grade malignancies that invade locally and only spread beyond the primary site in exceptional circumstances. It is felt that BCCs are derived from either follicular epithelium or undifferentiated basal layer cells. The tumour is comprised of darkly staining basaloid cells and shows characteristic palisading and clefting on pathological examination. BCCs are strongly associated with sun exposure, occurring more commonly on sun exposed sites and in patients with a large degree of cumulative sun exposure (e.g. outdoor workers). Up to two thirds of BCCs show a UV induced mutation in the PTCH gene which is part of the sonic hedgehog oncogene pathway.

**Table 7.1** Types of basal cell carcinoma

| Type of BCC | Clinical features |
| --- | --- |
| Nodular and nodulocystic BCC | The commonest presentation. A slow growing papule or nodule with a shiny appearance and telangiectasia, may mimic an intradermal naevus |
| Ulcerative BCC | When a nodular BCC outgrows its blood supply the centre becomes ischaemic and ulcerates. They present as an ulcer with well defined surrounding edge that has a pearly appearance and telangiectasia |
| Superficial BCC | Thin lesions that spread horizontally rather than vertically. They often have a non-specific appearance, presenting as a red patch |
| Pigmented BCC | An uncommon presentation of a nodular or ulcerative BCC with brown-black pigment. They are diagnostically challenging |
| Morphoeic/sclerosing BCC | Infiltrative BCCs that may resemble scar tissue or have a more typical BCC appearance. These BCCs often infiltrate well beyond the clinically discernable edge |
| Pinkus tumour | A rare variant of BCC presenting in elderly men with the appearance of a skin tag |

In this question the patient has a lesion clinically typical of a small basal cell carcinoma. Suitable treatments would include excision and radiotherapy. Given the patient's relatively young age excision with appropriate 4 mm margins would give a better cosmetic outcome than radiotherapy in the long run. As the lesion is primary, well defined, small and not adjacent to any vital structures Mohs micrographic surgery is not required. If curettage was to be performed three cycles would be required.

## 120 E. Excision of the skin graft and Mohs micrographic surgery to the whole site

Basal cell carcinoma is common and may be treated with a number of different modalities. Choosing the best treatment is dependent on the lesion type, size, location and the patient's age and health status.

Surgical excision is the treatment of choice for the majority of primary basal cell carcinomas. In experienced hands the recurrence rate of BCCs after excision with appropriate margins is less than 2% at 5 years. For most primary BCCs a peripheral excision margin of 4 mm and deep margin of subcutaneous fat is appropriate, although this will depend on the location and size of the BCC. It is recommended that large, morphoeic and recurrent BCCs have a wider surgical margin.

Mohs micrographic surgery is a technique whereby tumours are removed by staged excision and the surgical margins are examined completely. This allows for complete removal of BCCs with minimal loss of surrounding tissue. Cure rates for primary BCCs removed by this method are over 99%. Indications for Mohs micrographic surgery include:
- BCCs of the central face, especially those close to the eye
- large or morphoeic BCCs
- BCCs with poorly defined clinical margins
- recurrent or incompletely excised lesions.

Curettage and cautery (C&C) is an outdated technique that is heavily dependent on operator experience and careful lesion selection. A triple pass method is recommended where the lesion in both curetted and curettaged on three occasions. Even for selected low risk BCCs cure rates are less than 93%. C&C may be used as a primary treatment for small, well defined, non-facial BCCs in elderly patients. It also has a role in debulking tumours prior to other treatment modalities, for example radiotherapy.

Cryotherapy may be used in the treatment of certain low risk BCCs. It is a recognised and commonly used treatment for superficial BCC. When used for nodular or invasive BCCs the treatment is highly operator dependent and relies on careful lesion selection.

Radiotherapy is highly effective in the treatment for primary, incompletely excised and recurrent BCC and has cure rates of 90%. Superficial radiotherapy is used for lesions up to 6mm in depth, electron beam therapy is used for deeper lesions and brachytherapy may be used on curved surfaces. Multiple fraction techniques tend to be used as they have a better cosmetic outcome although single fraction radiotherapy may be appropriate in the very elderly. Certain areas such as the upper eyelid and bridge of the nose should be avoided due to the increased risk of radionecrosis.

Photodynamic therapy (PDT) involves the application of a photosensitising cream that is selectively taken up by tumour cells and then exposed to intense light that induced apoptosis. There is good evidence for the use of MAL-PDT in superficial BCCs with clearance rates of 97% at 3 months. When used for selected, thin nodular BCCs it is less effective with 91% clearance at 3 months. PDT is expensive and time consuming but offers a superior cosmetic outcome.

Imiquimod is an immune response modifier that is licensed for the treatment of superficial BCCs. When used topically 5 times per week for 6 weeks clearance rates approached 80%. Long term data on the use of imiquimod for nodular and invasive BCC is awaited.

In this question the patient is presenting with an incompletely excised BCC from the inner canthus that has been repaired with a skin graft. Given the proximity of the lesion to the orbit Mohs micrographic surgery is the treatment of choice. Even with the use of a marking suture there is always some uncertainty of the location of the involved margin and convention is to remove the whole graft and take a circumferential Mohs layer. Radiotherapy is technically possible but undesirable in such close proximity to the eye.

## 121 B. Lesion A requires re-excision, lesion B does not
Squamous cell carcinoma (SCC) is the second most common type of skin cancer and arises from the keratinising cells of the epidermis or its appendages. It has a variable appearance and may mimic a BCC, actinic keratosis or viral wart. SCCs are often ill-defined red lesions with a rough, scaly surface that may ulcerate, they may also present as a cutaneous horn. Rarely, they may present as a verrucous carcinoma, with a warty appearance on the hands, feet, anogenital area or buccal mucosa.

Risk factors for SCC include:
* chronic ultraviolet or ionising radiation exposure
* fair skin, albinism

- xeroderma pigmentosum
- immunosuppression, leukaemia, lymphoma, organ transplantation
- arsenic ingestion
- chronic wounds, ulcers, scars, burns, sinuses
- Bowen's disease (SCC in situ)
- biological agents (possibly)
- HPV infection.

SCCs are more aggressive than BCCs and if left untreated will metastasise. A number of SCC features are associated with metastatic potential and are used to classify lesions as low or high risk as shown in Table 7.2.

**Table 7.2** Low and high risk features of squamous cell carcinoma

| Low risk SCCs | High risk SCCs |
| --- | --- |
| • SCCs arising on sun exposed sites<br>• Less than 2 cm diameter<br>• Tumours less than 2 mm in thickness and confined to the upper dermis<br>• Well differentiated SCCs<br>• Verrucous subtype of SCCs<br>• Immunocompetent patient | • SCCs from the lip, ear, non-sun exposed sites, areas of chronic inflammation or injury<br>• Greater than 2 cm diameter<br>• Tumours greater than 4 mm in depth and invading the subcutaneous tissues<br>• Poorly differentiated SCCs<br>• Desmoplastic, acantholytic and spindle subtypes of SCCs<br>• SCCs with perineural, lymphatic or vascular invasion<br>• SCCs arising from an area of Bowen's (in situ) disease<br>• Immunosuppressed patients<br>• Recurrent/incompletely excised SCC |

Treatment of SCC is primarily surgical. Low risk SCCs should be removed with a 4–5 mm clinical margin and high risk SCCs should be removed with a 6–10 mm clinical margin. Ideally SCCs should be excised to the plane below subcutaneous fat, for example fascia. The exact clinical margin is dependent on the tumour size, local anatomy and patient frailty. Mohs micrographic surgery is useful in SCC and has similar indications as for BCC (*see* question 120). Curettage and cautery and cryosurgery should only be used by an experienced practitioner for small, well defined low risk SCCs. Radiotherapy is an effective treatment for SCCs and highly suitable for elderly patients.

In this question, lesion A should be considered high risk. Although well differentiated it has arisen within an area of Bowen's disease, it measures over 2 cm in diameter and invades over 4 mm into the deep dermis. It has been excised with a relatively narrow peripheral margin of 5 mm and a shallow deep margin of subcutaneous fat. This lesion should be re-excised to the depth of the aponeurosis and a cumulative peripheral margin of 7–10 mm. Lesion B can be considered low to medium risk. Although it is moderately differentiated, it is small, arising on a sun exposed site and only invades 2 mm into the upper dermis. The 7 mm peripheral margins and excision to the depth of the aponeurosis should be adequate for this lesion. Radiotherapy is not a good choice in this relatively young patient.

## 122 D. Excision biopsy

Keratoacanthomas are common skin tumours that occur on sun exposed sites. They occur suddenly and expand rapidly up to 2 cm in diameter over a few weeks. They clinically appear as a well defined nodule with a central keratin plug. After a number of weeks they spontaneously regress without sequelae. Pathologically and clinically they are similar in appearance to well differentiated SCCs with significant cytological atypia and a high mitotic rate. For a pathologist to confidently diagnose keratoacanthoma they need to examine the whole specimen to account for the overall architecture of the lesion. It is thought that up to 10% of lesions diagnosed as keratoacanthomas are actually well differentiated SCCs and many dermatologists feel that all keratoacanthomas should be treated as SCCs.

In this question the patient should undergo an excision biopsy with minimal surgical margins. With other forms of skin biopsy the pathologist will not be able to diagnose keratoacanthoma as they need to examine the architecture of the whole lesion. Radiotherapy should not be undertaken without a clear histological diagnosis. If the results of the excision biopsy are reported as an SCC further surgery or radiotherapy would be required.

## 123 B. Re-excision of 8mm around the scar

Melanoma is a less common type of skin cancer but it accounts for over 75% of skin cancer deaths. It typically presents as a new pigmented lesion or a pre-existing naevus that is expanding.

**Table 7.3** Subtypes of melanoma and their presentation

| Type of melanoma | Description |
|---|---|
| Melanoma in situ | A precursor to invasive melanoma, malignant melanoma cells are present but they do not show invasive growth. It presents with a similar appearance to a superficial spreading melanoma. Treatment is surgical excision with a margin to encompass any non-contiguous local dysplasia |
| Superficial spreading melanoma | The commonest presentation of melanoma often occurring on the backs of males and the legs of females as an enlarging, flat, irregular pigmented lesion. It may develop from a melanoma in situ or a dysplastic naevus. During this phase the melanoma is growing radially and tends to be thin with a good prognosis |
| Nodular melanoma | An aggressive form of melanoma that invades vertically leading to a thick lesion with a poor prognosis. It presents as an enlarging nodule that is often pigmented and may bleed |
| Acral lentiginous melanoma | Melanoma presenting on the sole, palm or subungually. It is the most common type of melanoma in pigmented racial groups. It presents later in life and is not related to sun exposure. Patients often present late and the prognosis is poor |
| Mucosal/eye melanoma | Melanomas that occur within the eye or on mucosal surfaces such as the vulva or bowel. These are rare and tend to present late |
| Desmoplastic melanoma | A rare histological subtype of melanoma that behaves aggressively |
| Amelanotic melanoma | A rare type of melanoma where melanin is not present. Lesions present as non-specific pink-red papules or nodules. They are often diagnosed late and carry a poor prognosis |
| Lentigo maligna | Occurs on sun damaged skin (e.g. face) in the elderly as an irregular pigmented macule/patch. Malignant melanoma cells are present but they do not show invasive growth. Treatment is surgical excision, if left untreated lentigo maligna melanoma may occur |
| Lentigo maligna melanoma | A melanoma that has occurred within a lentigo maligna, it often presents as a darkly pigmented papule or nodule within the pigmented patch |

Risk factors for melanoma include:
- pale skin type
- living in sunnier climates
- use of tanning salons

- multiple atypical or dysplastic naevi
- giant congenital naevus
- family history of melanoma.

When melanoma is suspected the lesion should be excised in full with a margin of 2 mm. This allows the pathologist to examine the overall architecture of the lesion and obtain an accurate measure of the lesion's Breslow thickness. In a few instances, such as lentigo maligna melanoma, an incisional biopsy may be taken but this must be interpreted with the greatest of care in view of the possibility of sampling error. Breslow thickness is a measure of the depth of tumour invasion using an ocular micrometer. It is a widely used measure that can be directly correlated to patient prognosis.

Once a diagnosis of primary melanoma has been established wide local surgical excision is undertaken, this is the only intervention that has a proven impact on patient prognosis. The diameter of the wide local excision is determined by the Breslow thickness of the tumour.

**Table 7.4** Breslow thickness of melanoma, 5-year survival and surgical margins required

| Breslow thickness | Stage | Approximate 5-year survival | Wide local excision surgical margin |
| --- | --- | --- | --- |
| 0 mm (in situ) | 0 | 99% | 2–5 mm |
| Less than 1 mm | I | 95–99% | 1 cm |
| 1–2 mm | I/II | 80–95% | 2 cm |
| 2.1–4 mm | II | 60–75% | 2–3 cm |
| Greater than 4 mm | II | 50% | 3 cm |

In this question the patient has had a 2 mm margin diagnostic excision of a thin, 0.2 mm melanoma. In accordance with guidelines a further 8 mm of tissue should be removed bringing the total excision margin to 1 cm. Radiotherapy has no place in the treatment of primary melanoma although it may be used for palliative treatment of metastatic disease.

### 124 D. Excision of the local cutaneous metastasis and block lymph node dissection in the groin

Metastatic melanoma should be managed by a multidisciplinary team of dermatologists, oncologists, surgeons, radiologists and pathologists. With appropriate treatment there is potential for long term survival or even cure.

Table 7.5 Staging and 5-year survival of metastatic melanoma

| Stage | Features | 5-year survival |
|-------|----------|-----------------|
| 0 | Melanoma in situ | 99% |
| I | Primary melanoma less than 1 mm Breslow with ulceration or less than 2 mm without ulceration | 85–95% |
| II | Primary melanoma greater than 1 mm Breslow with ulceration or greater than 2 mm without ulceration | 40–85% |
| III | Lymph node, regional or in transit metastasis | 25–60% |
| IV | Distant metastatic spread | 9–15% |

Investigations such as imaging should only be undertaken in patients with stage IIB disease and above due to a high rate of false positive results. Appropriate investigations include a chest X-ray, ultrasound of the liver or CT scan, liver function tests, serum LDH and a full blood count. There is no role for adjuvant treatment of melanoma although a number of clinical trials are being undertaken in this area. Isolated limb perfusion may have a role as a neoadjuvant treatment to reduce tumour volume prior to surgery. The role of sentinel lymph node biopsy in melanoma is yet to be established and it should only be undertaken within a registered clinical trial.

Patients with suspected metastatic regional lymphadenopathy should undergo fine needle aspiration cytology of the enlarged node(s). If metastatic regional lymphadenopathy is confirmed the patient should undergo a radical block lymph node dissection by an experienced melanoma surgeon. If relapse occurs in further lymph node basins block dissection should be performed. Post-operative radiotherapy may have a role in reducing recurrence if a block lymph node dissection is incomplete.

Local, regional and solitary distant metastases should be treated surgically with narrow margin excision. Isolated limb perfusion/ infusion regional chemotherapy is used for multiple loco-regional metastases in a limb. Radiotherapy has a role in the palliation of symptomatic disease but does not alter prognosis. Patients with stage IV disease may be considered for chemotherapy either with dacarbazine or as part of a clinical trial.

In this question a young woman is presenting with loco-regional recurrence of a thick melanoma from her leg. Appropriate treatment would be excision of the local metastasis and block lymph node dissection of the groin by an experienced melanoma surgeon. Selective removal of enlarged lymph nodes would be unsatisfactory due to the likelihood of micrometastasis in other local lymph nodes. There is no role for radiotherapy or isolated limb infusion in the patient at this stage.

## 125 A. Dermatofibrosarcoma protuberans

Dermatofibrosarcoma protuberans (DFSP) is a rare malignant fibrohistiocytic tumour with significant potential for local recurrence. It presents in young or middle-aged adults as a slowly growing dermal plaque or nodule that may enter a rapid growth phase. Most cases show a t(17;22) chromosomal translocation that fuses the platelet-derived growth factor gene with the collagen 1 gene. Treatment is with wide local excision or Mohs micrographic surgery. Local recurrence occurs in up to 30% of cases, distant metastatic spread occurs in less than 5% of cases.

Merkel cell carcinoma is a rare and highly aggressive neuroendocrine tumour of the skin. It presents as a rapidly growing, painless, firm nodule that may be skin coloured, red or blue. It is most commonly seen in elderly Caucasians but may be seen in any ethnic group. The newly identified Merkel cell polyomavirus seems to play a key role in the aetiology of the cancer. Treatment of primary disease is wide local excision with or without radiotherapy; metastatic disease is treated with chemotherapy.

Angiosarcoma is another rare and highly aggressive type of skin cancer. It is derived from the cells of blood vessel endothelium. Risk factors for angiosarcoma include longstanding lymphoedema, radiotherapy, arsenic, vinyl chloride and longstanding foreign body reactions. Cutaneous angiosarcomas often present on the head and neck of elderly patients as an enlarging bruise or vascular nodule. Treatment is wide local excision with or without radiotherapy. Prognosis is often poor.

Liposarcomas are rare soft tissue tumours that often present in the thigh or retroperitoneum. Prognosis is dependent on the histological subtype of the tumour.

Kaposi's sarcoma see question 135.

In this question the patient is presenting with a malignant fibrohistiocytic tumour most likely to be a dermatofibrosarcoma protuberans.

## 126 C. Mohs micrographic surgery

In this question the patient is presenting with an atypical fibroxanthoma (AFX). It is a rare skin tumour that is most often seen on the head and neck of elderly patients. Cumulative sun exposure and previous radiotherapy are risk factors for developing AFX. It presents as a red, juicy dome shaped nodule that may be crusty or ulcerated. They rapidly grow over 6–12 months enlarging to 2–3 cm in size. Histology shows fibrocystic, spindle-shaped and anaplastic cells with characteristic lipid containing multinucleated giant cells. The tumour is malignant and has the potential to metastasise but this is rare. The treatment of choice is surgery with a minimal margin.

In this case the patient has had a diagnostic excision of a large AFX. The minimal deep margin of 0.5 mm is concerning and a further excision would be appropriate. Mohs micrographic surgery would be the treatment of choice as this would allow for complete excision with maximum preservation on non-involved tissue.

## 127 C. Mammogram

Cutaneous deposits of internal malignancy are not uncommon and present as non-specific mobile nodules that may ulcerate. The deposits often occur late in the disease and are associated with a poor prognosis with an average life expectancy of 3–6 months. The commonest cause of cutaneous metastases in men is lung cancer and in women it is breast cancer. The scalp is a common site for metastases, most notably for breast, lung and gastrointestinal cancers. Renal carcinoma may metastasise to the mouth. Prostate cancer may present with an unusual zoster-like distribution after perineural and lymphatic spread.

In this question a middle-aged woman is presenting with a cutaneous deposit of adenocarcinoma on the scalp. The commonest cause of cutaneous metastases in women is breast carcinoma; therefore the most relevant investigation would be a mammogram.

## 128 D. Gastroenterology

Muir-Torre syndrome is a subtype of Lynch type II hereditary nonpolyposis colon cancer. It is due to an autosomal dominantly inherited mutation in DNA mismatch repair genes. Patients may present with sebaceous adenomas, sebaceous epitheliomas, sebaceous carcinoma, keratoacanthomas and basal cell carcinoma. These individuals have a significantly raised risk of visceral malignancy in particular colorectal carcinoma. Sebaceous gland tumours are rare in the general population and the finding of such a tumour should always prompt suspicion of Muir-Torre syndrome.

**Table 7.6** Congenital syndromes of malignancy with cutaneous features

| Syndrome | Cutaneous features | Malignancies seen |
|---|---|---|
| Gardner's syndrome | Epidermal cysts, lipomas, fibromas | Gastrointestinal, thyroid |
| Peutz-Jeghers syndrome | Mucocutaneous pigmentation | Gastrointestinal, pancreas, other |
| Howel-Evans syndrome | Palmoplantar keratoderma (tylosis) | Oesophageal |
| Muir-Torre syndrome | Sebaceous tumours, keratoacanthoma, BCC | Colorectal, other |
| Cowden syndrome | Trichilemmomas, mucosal warty hyperplasia | Breast, thyroid, endometrial, renal, other |
| Neurofibromatosis | Café-au-lait macules, neurofibromas, freckling | Schwannoma, glioma, leukaemia, CNS tumours, sarcoma |
| Tuberous sclerosis | Angiofibromas, periungual fibromas, shagreen patches | Sarcoma, rhabdomyoma, renal, angiomyolipoma |
| Gorlin syndrome | Multiple BCCs, palmar pits, typical facies | Medulloblastoma, breast, lymphoma |
| Von Hippel-Lindau disease | Cafe-au-lait, haemangiomas | Haemangioblastoma, renal, phaeochromocytoma |
| Wiskott-Aldridge syndrome | Eczema | Lymphoma, leukaemia |

In this question a patient is presenting with multiple sebaceous tumours, given the family history the most likely diagnosis is Muir-Torre syndrome. Such patients should be referred to a gastroenterologist due to the high incidence of colorectal carcinoma.

### 129 E. Acute myeloid leukaemia

Sweet's syndrome is a rare dermatosis strongly associated with internal malignancy. Patients present with plum coloured papules and plaques, fever and leukocytosis. Histology is of a dense neutrophilic infiltrate throughout the dermis sometimes extending to the subcutis, vasculitic changes may also be present. There is a strong association with malignancy, in particular haematological malignancies, and collagen-vascular disorders. Treatment is with systemic corticosteroids.

**Table 7.7** Cutaneous conditions associated with internal malignancy

| Cutaneous disorder | Associated malignancy |
| --- | --- |
| Dermatomyositis | 27% have malignancy – ovarian, breast, lung, gastrointestinal |
| Acanthosis nigricans | Gastrointestinal (poor prognostic indicator) |
| Necrolytic migratory erythema | Glucagonoma |
| Herpes zoster | Leukaemia, lymphoma |
| Seborrhoeic keratosis | Leser-Trelat sign – gastrointestinal, cutaneous lymphoma, leukaemia, lung, breast |
| Sweet's syndrome | Leukaemia, lymphoma |
| Erythroderma | Cutaneous lymphoma, Sézary's syndrome, leukaemia, lymphoma |
| Xanthomas | Multiple myeloma, haematological malignancies |
| Paraneoplastic pemphigus | Lymphoma |
| Erythema gyratum repens | Lung, gastrointestinal, breast |
| Flushing | Carcinoid syndrome, mastocytosis, phaeochromocytoma |
| Palmar erythema | Liver primary or metastases |
| Telangiectasia | Cutaneous deposits of internal malignancy, biliary tract tumours |
| Purpura | Lymphoma, leukaemia, myeloma |
| Superficial/migratory erythema | Pancreatic – also pruritus and nodular panniculitis |
| Acanthosis palmaris | Lung |
| Pruritus | Lymphoma, other |
| Acquired hypertrichosis lanuginosa | Gastrointestinal, lung – sign of late disease |
| Acquired ichthyosis | Lymphoma |
| Pyoderma gangrenosum | Haematological malignancies |
| Finger clubbing | Lung, cardiac |
| Pallor | Anything invading the bone marrow e.g. leukaemia |
| Diffuse hyperpigmentation | Ectopic ACTH from e.g. oat cell carcinoma of the lung |
| Erythema multiforme | Leukaemia, lymphoma |
| Dermatitis herpetiformis-like eruption | Rarely with some cancers |

In this question the patient has a rash and histology consistent with Sweet's syndrome. This disorder is particularly associated with haematological malignancies such as acute myeloid leukaemia.

### 130 B. Bexarotene

Mycosis fungoides is a rare, low-grade, primarily CD4-positive primary cutaneous lymphoma of the skin. It presents as persistent, treatment resistant scaly patches on the skin. There is often a significant delay in diagnosis with multiple non-diagnostic skin biopsies. Over time the skin patches thicken to become plaques and tumours, in late stage disease the lymph nodes and viscera are involved. Variants of mycosis fungoides include the following.

Small-plaque parapsoriasis (digitate dermatosis) – chronic annular, scaly plaques in a pityriasis rosea type distribution. Most cases do not progress to mycosis fungoides.

Large-plaque parapsoriasis – larger plaques often on the lower abdomen and upper legs, may be reticulate with telangiectasia (retiform parapsoriasis). Twenty per cent of cases progress to mycosis fungoides.

Granulomatous slack skin disease – a rare form of mycosis fungoides presenting as lax erythematous skin forming large pendulous folds.

Pagetoid reticulosis – single or grouped hyperkeratotic skin lesions that respond well to radiotherapy.

Sézary syndrome – a more aggressive form of mycosis fungoides in which patients present with erythroderma, lymphadenopathy and circulating Sézary cells (atypical mononuclear cells).

In addition to the classical patch/plaque/tumour forms of mycosis fungoides, other forms may present as follicular papules, pustules, alopecia, bullae, erythroderma, pigmentary change, vasculitis or hyperkeratosis.

There are a number of treatment options for mycosis fungoides depending on the stage of the disease.
• Topical therapies are used in early stage disease. They include topical steroids and nitrogen mustard.
• Light therapy is used when topical treatments fail, PUVA is more effective than UVB.
• Total skin electron beam therapy is a form of superficial total body radiotherapy, it is generally used third line for widespread cutaneous disease that does not respond to light therapy.

- Radiotherapy is an effective treatment of problematic areas such as an ulcerating cutaneous tumour.
- Alfa-interferon, bexarotene, methotrexate, alemtuzumab and denileukin diftitox are systemic agents used when there is treatment resistant cutaneous disease or lymphadenopathy.
- Extracorporeal photopheresis is used as a first line treatment in Sézary syndrome and is effective for advanced mycosis fungoides.
- Chemotherapy is used for erythrodermic patients or those with systemic involvement or treatment resistant advanced disease.

In this question bexarotene therapy would be inappropriate for early-stage mycosis fungoides. Primary treatments would be topical corticosteroids, nitrogen mustard and light therapy. Secondary treatments could include alpha-interferon and total skin electron beam therapy.

## 131 A. Chronic lymphocytic leukaemia

Chronic lymphocytic leukaemia (CLL) is the commonest cause of leukaemia cutis. It may present as papules, nodules, plaques, erythema or bullae. The face and extremities are the commonest sites for leukaemia cutis and it may show koebnerization. When CLL infiltrates the face it may result in a leonine facies or a rosacea-like eruption. Myeloid line leukaemia cutis tends to present on the trunk as red-purple papules, plaques or nodules that may ulcerate. Myelomonocytic disease can cause gingival hyperplasia. A chloroma is a green coloured deposit of leukaemic cells, often myeloid in origin in the skin.

Systemic lymphomas rarely infiltrate the skin. When they do the lesions are non-specific and may present as pruritus, pigmentary change, ichthyosis, alopecia or exfoliative dermatitis.

Primary B-cell lymphomas of the skin are rare, often presenting as a single purple nodule they are treated with radiotherapy. Approximately 10% are associated with Borrelia Burgdorferi infection.

Lymphomatoid papulosis is a chronic skin eruption of self-healing papulonodules that crust, ulcerate and heal with atrophic scarring. Twenty per cent of patients with lymphomatoid papulosis either have or subsequently develop lymphoma.

## 132 A. Inability to raise the forehead on the ipsilateral side and possible ptosis

Nerve damage during dermatological surgery is rare but there are a small number of nerves that run superficially and may be affected.

The temporal branch of the facial nerve passes superficially over the zygomatic arch in the temple region and supplies parts of the frontalis, obicularis oculi and corrugator supercilii muscles. Damage to the nerve can lead to an inability to raise the ipsilateral forehead and contribute to a ptosis.

The marginal mandibular branch of the facial nerve passes forward beneath the platysma and triangularis and crosses the mandible and supplies the muscles of the lower lip and chin. Damage to the nerve can lead to drooping of the ipsilateral lip, drooling and an asymmetrical smile.

The distal motor component of the spinal accessory nerve is prone to damage as it pierces the sternocleidomastoid muscle at Erb's point in the posterior triangle of the neck. Paralysis of the trapezius muscle may ensue leading to winging of the scapula and difficulty abducting the arm.

Any surgery below the subcutis of the forehead risks damage to the superficial branches of the supraorbital and supratrochlear nerves. These nerves supply sensation to the forehead.

The sural nerve may be damaged during lower limb surgery. It runs superficially down the posterior calf to the lateral malleolus. It is a sensory nerve and damage leads to loss of sensation to the posterolateral calf, lateral ankle and lateral plantar foot.

In this question damage to the temporal branch of the facial nerve may lead to an inability to raise the ipsilateral forehead and contribute to a ptosis.

### 133 C. 50 mls

The maximum safe dose of plain lignocaine in an adult is 3 mg/kg, with adrenalin up to 7 mg/kg may be used. In children and the elderly these doses should be halved. 1% lignocaine has 10 mg/ml.

**Table 7.8** Features of lignocaine toxicity

| Time | Symptoms and signs |
| --- | --- |
| Early | Light headedness, dizziness, tinnitus, circumoral numbness, abnormal taste, confusion, drowsiness |
| Late | Tonic-clonic convulsions, loss of consciousness, coma, respiratory depression, respiratory arrest, cardiovascular collapse, arrhythmias |

In this question a 70 kg adult may be given up to 7 mg/kg of lignocaine with adrenalin. This equates to 490 mg, or 49 mls of 1% solution.

## 134 D. Minocycline treatment

Acanthosis nigricans is a rash of velvety hyperpigmentation seen most commonly in the axillae. It is often associated with skin tags and may occur in other sites such as the neck, groin, mouth, hands and perianal region. Histologically it shows hyperkeratosis, acanthosis and papillomatosis.

Pseudo-acanthosis nigricans is most commonly seen in association with obesity and endocrine disorders such as diabetes and Cushing's disease. It is thought that friction and maceration of the flexures plays a role in the disorder's aetiology.

Congenital acanthosis nigricans is inherited in an autosomal dominant manner. The rash often appears before puberty and may be associated with mental retardation and neurofibromatosis.

True acanthosis nigricans is rare, it presents in non-obese adults and is always associated with cancer. It is a poor prognostic sign usually associated with disseminated disease. Mouth and hand (triple palm) lesions are characteristic.

In this question endocrine disorders and malignancy are both associated with acanthosis nigricans. Minocycline is not a known association although it may cause hyperpigmentation.

## 135 E. Individuals who have previously received radiotherapy treatment

Kaposi's sarcoma (KS) is a mixed spindle cell and vascular tumour caused by infection with human herpes virus 8 (HHV8). It presents as lesions that may be red, purple, brown or black; often papular it may also present as macules, nodules, patches, plaques or tumours. The surface may be scaly, ulcerated or haemorrhagic and the lesions show koebnerization. A number of subtypes of KS have been described.

Classical KS affects elderly men of Eastern European, Mediterranean and Ashkenazi Jewish descent. It is an indolent disease that often starts around the toes and soles and coalesces into nodules and plaques. It is thought that this form of KS may be a hyperplasia rather than a true neoplasia.

AIDS associated KS is an aggressive disease presenting with rapidly progressive Kaposi's lesions that may be fatal without treatment. KS is over 20 times more common in HIV infected individuals and is also more common in homosexual males due to prevalence of HHV8 infection.

Endemic or African cutaneous KS presents in young adults from tropical and sub-Saharan Africa. It is an aggressive form of KS affecting the lower limbs with progressive cutaneous disease.

African lymphadenopathic KS occurs in children under 10 years of age in Africa; it affects the lymph nodes with or without cutaneous involvement and is often fatal.

Transplant or immunosuppression related KS presents in a similar manner to classical KS and is associated with calcineurin inhibitors such as ciclosporin.

Treatment of KS may be with surgery, radiotherapy, interferon or chemotherapy. KS cannot be cured but may be palliated for many years in a similar manner to mycosis fungoides. In patients with immunosuppression or HIV related KS restoration of immune function often leads to rapid KS remission.

In this question groups at risk of developing Kaposi's sarcoma include those with HIV infection, homosexual males, elderly Africans and Ashkenazi Jews. Homosexual males without HIV are at significantly higher risk of HHV8 infection and predisposition to develop Kaposi's sarcoma. Previous radiotherapy is a risk factor for angiosarcoma not Kaposi's sarcoma.

## 136 E. Hyperthyroidism

Xanthomas are due to cutaneous deposits of lipid laden macrophages and they occur in patients with an abnormality of lipid metabolism. They may present in a number of ways.

Xanthelasma are yellow plaques that occur around the eyes and are associated with increased risk of cardiovascular disease. Most patients have normal lipid and cholesterol levels and are thought to have other abnormalities in apolipoprotein metabolism.

Eruptive xanthomas present as multiple small yellow-brown papules that occur in crops on the buttocks, thighs and elbows. They are associated with very high triglyceride levels and carry risks of pancreatitis and type-2 diabetes. They may also be associated with monoclonal gammaopathy.

Tuberous xanthomas are larger and deeper, occurring as nodules in the subcutis. Associated with high cholesterol levels and increased cardiovascular risk they may be attached to tendons.

Xanthomas may occur as a secondary phenomenon related to other disorders, such as:
- hyperlipidaemia syndrome

- diabetes and impaired glucose tolerance
- obesity
- alcohol abuse
- oestrogens, retinoids, ritonavir
- cholestasis – biliary atresia, haemochromatosis, primary biliary cirrhosis
- hypothyroidism
- nephrotic syndrome
- gammopathies.

In this question hyperthyroidism is not a recognised cause of xanthomas although hypothyroidism is.

## 137 D. The oral contraceptive pill

The description is of a spider naevus, also called a spider angioma or a naevus araneus. These are common, benign, acquired vascular lesions present in over 10% of healthy adults. They typically occur in the distribution of the superior vena cava, that is the face, neck, upper chest and upper arms. During pregnancy they often occur and spontaneously resolve postpartum. Treatment is either with electrodesiccation or laser.

Causes of spider naevi:

- pregnancy
- the oral contraceptive pill
- liver disease.

Spider naevi are not associated with prematurity, although they are more common in children and women. Sturge-Weber syndrome is a congenital arteriovenous malformation leading to a facial port wine stain and intracranial abnormalities.

## 138 A. Isotretinoin

Keloid scars are formed due to overgrowth of granulation tissue at a site of skin injury and they are composed of type III and type I collagen. They present as firm, rubbery, non-tender nodules that may hyperpigment. Often they are pruritic and may be painful. They should be distinguished from hypertrophic scars.

**Table 7.9** Key features of hypertrophic and keloid scars

|  | Hypertrophic scars | Keloid scars |
|---|---|---|
| Clinical features | Red, raised, firm and often pruritic the scars do not extend beyond the site of initial trauma and flatten with time | More exaggerated than hypertrophic scars they extend beyond the borders of the original trauma and only rarely involute |
| Demographics | All races, not familial, any age but often children | Increased risk in Afro-Caribbeans and Asians, may be familial, most common in young adults |
| History | Tend to occur within 2 months of injury | Tend to occur within 1 month of injury |
| Site | May occur at any site | Increased risk at sites of tensioned skin and over bony prominences |
| Treatment | May be surgically corrected | Surgery may worsen the scar, medical treatment with steroids, silicone gel, compression or radiation |

Risk factors for developing a keloid scar include:
- family or personal history of keloids
- Afro-Caribbean or Asian ethnicity
- thermal injuries
- high risk sites (*see* above)
- isotretinoin therapy
- rare genodermatosis – Ehlers-Danlos syndrome, osteogenesis imperfecta, progeria.

In this question the patient would be at greater risk of developing a keloid scar if they were taking isotretinoin.

### 139 D. Antihelix

Chondrodermatitis nodularis helicis (CNH) is a common, benign, inflammatory condition of the ear. It classically presents in middle-aged and elderly men, although it also occurs in women and the young. A rapidly enlarging painful nodule appears on the ear and enlarges to its maximum size where it remains stable. The nodule may have a rolled edge and central ulcer or crust. They are more common on the right ear and are occasionally seen bilaterally. In men it is most often seen on the superior helix, in women the antihelix is most often affected. Patients often sleep on the affected side. CNH may be precipitated by pressure damage, cold, actinic damage and repeated trauma. Treatment is with pressure relieving devices such as special pillows, topical or intralesional steroids or a variety of surgical/destructive methods.

In this question the commonest site for CNH in women is the antihelix, in men it is the superior helix.

# Chapter 8

# Paediatric dermatology and genodermatology

## QUESTIONS

**140** A one-day-old baby is referred with an extensive flat, vascular patch covering most of the left side of the face. It extends from the mandible to the forehead, laterally to the ear and medially to the nasal bridge. What investigation should be organised as a matter of urgency:

A  CT scan of the head and neck
B  MRI of the brain
C  ophthalmology review
D  ultrasound of the face
E  an EEG.

**141** You are asked to review a well one-year-old child with a lesion on her cheek. On examination there is an intact 3 cm red nodule consistent with a superficial haemangioma over the lateral right cheek. What treatment is appropriate:

A  do nothing
B  topical potent corticosteroid
C  intralesional injection with corticosteroid
D  laser
E  embolisation.

**142** A 12-year-old boy is referred by his general practitioner with 'eczema'. On examination he has large, firmly adherent brown scales consistent with an ichthyosis. His parents have normal skin, but his maternal grandfather had a similar condition. What is the most likely diagnosis:

A   ichthyosis vulgaris
B   epidermolytic hyperkeratosis
C   lamellar ichthyosis
D   steroid sulphatase deficiency
E   congenital ichthyosiform erythroderma.

**143** You are asked to see a newborn baby born with a collodion membrane. The child's parents wish to know the prognosis, which of the following is most accurate:

A   the membrane will not resolve, there is a 100% chance of ichthyosis
B   the membrane will resolve in 2–3 weeks, 60% chance of ichthyosis
C   the membrane will resolve in 6 months, 100% chance of ichthyosis
D   the membrane will resolve in 6 months, 50% chance of ichthyosis
E   the membrane will resolve in 2–3 weeks, less than 10% chance of ichthyosis.

**144** A 16-year-old boy presents with greasy papules and plaques in seborrhoeic areas consistent with Darier's disease. He mentions that other members of his family have this condition. What is the mode of inheritance of Darier's disease:

A   autosomal recessive
B   autosomal dominant
C   x-linked recessive
D   x-linked dominant
E   not genetically inherited.

**145** A four-year-old girl is seen in the neurology clinic with a recent onset of seizures. You are asked to review her as she has a number of hypopigmented patches on her skin. Under Wood's light the patches are highlighted and you suspect a diagnosis of tuberous sclerosis. Which of the following is not a feature of tuberous sclerosis:

A   precocious puberty
B   periungual fibromas
C   retinal phakoma
D   psychiatric illness
E   dental enamel pits.

**146** A 10-day-old baby boy is referred with multiple brown marks on his body. On examination the baby has 14 light brown, well defined patches consistent with café au lait macules. In which of the following disorders are numerous café au lait macules not a feature:

A   tuberous sclerosis
B   neurofibromatosis
C   ataxia telangiectasia
D   McCune-Albright syndrome
E   Ehlers-Danlos syndrome.

**147** A patient is seen with hyperextensible skin and joints suspicious of Ehlers-Danlos syndrome. What key protein is abnormal in most cases of Ehlers-Danlos syndrome:

A   elastin
B   collagen
C   mucin
D   fibrin
E   keratin.

**148** A 15-year-old patient is referred with thickened yellow skin on her neck. On further examination she has a similar appearance of bumpy, lax, yellow skin in the groins and flexures. She says that she has a distant relative with a similar condition who died young from a myocardial infarction. What is the most likely diagnosis:

A   cutis laxa
B   Marfan syndrome
C   epidermolysis bullosa simplex
D   psuedoxanthoma elasticum
E   Ehlers-Danlos syndrome.

**149** A 12-year-old girl presents with fragile skin, blisters and palmar-plantar keratoderma. The blisters have an unusual herpetiform grouping. Her mother says that soon after birth she was extremely unwell with widespread severe blistering. You suspect epidermolysis bullosa, what type is the patient most likely to have:

A   Weber-Cockayne
B   Herlitz junctional
C   non-Herlitz junctional
D   recessive dystrophic
E   Dowling-Meara.

**150** A young patient from an African family presents at birth with white skin, red hair and nystagmus. What is the most common mode of inheritance for this disorder:

A   autosomal recessive
B   autosomal dominant
C   x-linked recessive
D   x-linked dominant
E   not genetically inherited.

**151** A young child is under the care of the neurology team with progressive cerebellar dysfunction and is referred to you because of skin changes. On examination the child has numerous telangiectasia visible on the skin and eyes. What is the likely diagnosis:

A   CREST syndrome
B   telangiectasia macularis eruptiva perstans
C   ataxia telangiectasia
D   generalised essential telangiectasia
E   hereditary haemorrhagic telangiectasia.

**152** You review a four-month-old baby girl with severe eczema. Despite treatment with medium potency topical steroids she continues to have severe eczema on her face and buttocks and she has mild alopecia. What investigation would be most relevant for this patient:

A   patch testing to medicaments
B   total serum IgE level
C   specific IgE levels
D   prick testing to common allergens
E   serum zinc level.

**153** A seven-month-old baby is referred by their general practitioner with a sore rash in the nappy area. On examination the child is unkempt and the nappy is soiled, there is confluent erythema with scaling under the nappy but sparing of the groin folds. There are no satellite lesions and the rest of the skin, hair and nails are normal. What is the most likely cause of this rash:

A   psoriasis
B   irritant contact dermatitis
C   allergic contact dermatitis
D   atopy
E   candidal infection.

**154** Which of the following is not a feature of ectodermal dysplasia:

A   cleft palate
B   hyperhidrosis
C   hypopigmentation
D   absent teeth
E   dystrophic finger nails.

**155** A two-year-old child is referred by their general practitioner with a widespread rash that has followed an upper respiratory tract infection. On examination the child has a rash consisting of small, pink, flat topped monomorphic papules symmetrically involving the face, buttocks and extremities. It is not particularly itchy. What treatment would you recommend:

A   aciclovir syrup for 10 days
B   erythromycin syrup for 7 days
C   topical 1% hydrocortisone ointment twice daily
D   prednisolone 1 mg/kg tapering over 2 weeks
E   bland emollients.

**156** Which of the following is a common feature of Marfan's syndrome:

A   downwards dislocation of the lens
B   skin fragility
C   low, wide arched palate
D   scarring alopecia
E   striae.

**157** A two-year-old child is referred with a number of lesions on the skin. When one of these lesions get irritated it swells up and becomes urticated. You suspect a diagnosis of mastocytosis. Which of the following features carries the worst prognosis for this condition:

A   bullous skin lesions
B   numerous skin lesions
C   mast cells circulating in peripheral blood
D   mast cells in the bone marrow
E   raised serum mast cell tryptase enzyme.

**158** Which of the following is not a typical feature of multifocal unisystem Langerhans cell histiocytosis:

A   hepatosplenomegaly
B   osteolytic bone lesions
C   seborrhoeic dermatitis-like rash
D   skin ulcers
E   pathological fractures.

**159** Which of the following is pathological when seen in a newborn:

A   vernix caseosa
B   cutis marmorata
C   milia
D   miliaria crystalline
E   aplasia cutis.

**160** A one-day-old baby presents with a widespread rash of blotchy erythematous macules with central vesicles. You suspect a diagnosis of erythema toxicum neonatorum. The baby's mother asks when the rash will resolve, what is the correct answer:

A   within a few hours
B   within 24 hours
C   up to 5 days
D   2–3 weeks
E   over a month.

**161** You are called to the neonatal unit to review an unwell newborn baby. The baby has numerous red-blue papules and nodules on their skin consistent with a blueberry muffin baby. Which of the following is a cause of this presentation:

A   congenital herpes simplex infection
B   congenital tuberculosis infection
C   trisomy 13
D   congenital cytomegalovirus infection
E   congenital syphilis infection.

**162** You review a one-week-old child who has been referred with a subcutaneous nodule on the back. You suspect subcutaneous fat necrosis of the newborn, which blood test should be performed:

A   calcium
B   zinc
C   transaminase
D   full blood count
E   lipase.

## ANSWERS

### 140 C. Ophthalmology review

Port wine stains are flat vascular birthmarks present at birth. Most commonly seen on the face they rarely cross the midline and are often dermatomal. As patients get older the port wine stain may hypertrophy and become more cosmetically disfiguring. Treatment is with laser which is often given at the age of 1 to 2 years. Sturge-Weber syndrome is characterised by the presence of a V1/V2 trigeminal port wine stain and one or more of a number of abnormalities:

- ipsilateral meningeal and/or cerebral vascular malformation
- intracranial calcification
- seizures
- hemiplegia
- glaucoma
- mental retardation
- oral/lip hypertrophy.

A salmon patch is another common congenital vascular lesion. Most often seen on the forehead, glabellar and neck they present as a dull pink-red patch with telangiectasia. Salmon patches fade with time and do not need treatment. Fifty per cent of lesions in the nuchal region do persist but are often covered by hair.

In this question the patient has an extensive port wine stain and is likely to have Sturge-Weber syndrome. At this age assessment of neurological involvement will not alter management and does not need to be undertaken urgently. An early ophthalmology opinion is vital as the child may have glaucoma which would require treatment.

### 141 A. Do nothing

Haemangiomas are benign vascular malformations that rapidly enlarge over the first year of life. Typically it involutes from two years of age. They are classified as superficial (strawberry), deep (cavernous) or mixed. Haemangiomas occur more frequently in girls and premature babies. Rarely, if a haemangioma involves bone there may be osteolysis and fibrous replacement. Very large haemangiomas may cause destruction of platelets leading to thrombocytopenia, the Kasabach-Merritt syndrome. As haemangiomas spontaneously involute they are only treated if they are causing functional disturbance, for example covering an eye, or are bleeding. Treatments include steroids, laser, interferon, surgery, embolisation and beta-blockers. A number of syndromes exist in which multiple haemangiomas are seen as shown in Table 8.1.

**Table 8.1** Multiple haemangioma syndromes

| Name | Clinical features |
|---|---|
| Maffucci's syndrome | Haemangiomas, lymphangiomas, dyschondroplasia, bony and neurological abnormalities |
| Blue rubber bleb syndrome | Multiple haemangiomas on the skin and within internal organs |
| Cobb syndrome | Haemangioma or port wine stain on the back and a vascular malformation of the spinal cord |

In this question the patient has a medium sized superficial haemangioma on the lateral cheek. Appropriate treatment would be observation, allowing the haemangioma to naturally involute. Any active intervention risks scarring, topical steroids and laser are not required as the lesion is not bleeding. In the future patients such as this are likely to be given propranolol, but currently the results of large scale randomised control trials are awaited.

**142 D. Steroid sulphatase deficiency**
The ichthyosis are a family of skin disorders characterised by thick, scaly, flaky, dry skin. Most of the ichthyosis are congenital although rarely they may be acquired (*see* question 25). Treatment is with emollients and keratolytics, in severe cases acitretin may be helpful. Common and important ichthyosis include the following.

Ichthyosis vulgaris is a commonly seen autosomal dominant condition. Patients present with xerosis most prominent on the legs, fine powdery scale, accentuated palmar/plantar creases and pruritus.

Steroid sulphatase deficiency (X-linked ichthyosis) leads to a thickened epidermis and ichthyosis. Males present with prominent, dirty-brown, firmly adherent scales on the face, back and extensors. Sometimes described as fish scale the scalp is often affected and corneal opacities may occur. Female carriers may have a mild phenotype. Diagnosis can be made on serum cholesterol sulphatase levels.

Epidermolytic hyperkeratosis presents with large flaccid blisters in infancy and by the second decade patients develop erythematous, malodorous hyperkeratosis and verrucous plaques. It is due to a keratin mutation and may be spontaneous (50%) or inherited in an autosomal dominant fashion (50%).

Lamellar ichthyosis and non-bullous congenital ichthyosiform erythroderma (NBCIE) are severe ichthyosis inherited in an autosomal recessive manner. Patients present with a collodion membrane at birth then develop large, thick scales with fissuring, ectropion, scarring alopecia and nail abnormalities. NBCIE is milder than lamellar ichthyosis, it is less scaly and more erythrodermic.

Harlequin ichthyosis is very rare and often fatal in infancy. Children are born with thick, fissured plaques of skin, marked ectropion, eclabium and distorted flat ears. Difficulties include poor feeding, temperature and electrolyte regulation.

**Table 8.2** Ichthyosis 'plus' syndromes

| Name | Clinical features |
| --- | --- |
| Carvajal syndrome | Cardiomyopathy, woolly hair, keratoderma |
| CHILD Syndrome | Congenital hemidysplasia, ichthyosiform erythroderma, limb defects |
| Conradi-Hünermann syndrome | Bony deformities, growth retardation, facies, cataracts, erythroderma |
| Erythrokeratodermia variabilis | Generalised persistent brown hyperkeratosis with accentuated skin markings |
| IFAP syndrome | Ichthyosis follicularis, alopecia, and photophobia |
| Keratitis-ichthyosis-deafness syndrome | Progressive corneal opacification, either mild generalised hyperkeratosis or discrete erythematous plaques, and neurosensory deafness |
| Netherton syndrome | Trichorrhexis invaginata, erythroderma, allergies, Ichthyosis linearis circumflexa |
| Neutral lipid storage disease | Accumulation of triglycerides in the cytoplasm of leukocytes, muscle, liver, fibroblasts, and other tissues |
| Refsum's disease | Neurologic damage, cerebellar degeneration, peripheral neuropathy, night blindness, ataxia, ichthyosis and deafness |
| Rud syndrome | Night blindness, ataxia, ichthyosis, deafness, and eye problems |
| Sjögren-Larsson syndrome | Neurological problems, ichthyosis, mental retardation |
| Trichothiodystrophy | Congenital ichthyosiform erythroderma, growth retardation, mental retardation, progeria-like facies and brittle hair |

In this question the patient has steroid sulphatase deficiency, also known as x-linked ichthyosis. Ichthyosis vulgaris and epidermolytic hyperkeratosis are unlikely as his parents are unaffected and these conditions have an autosomal dominant inheritance. The patient also lacks the severe features of lamellar ichthyosis or non-bullous congenital ichthyosiform erythroderma.

### 143 B. The membrane will resolve in 2–3 weeks, 60% chance of ichthyosis

A collodion membrane is a transparent, parchment-like layer covering the skin at birth that desquamatises at 2–3 weeks of age. The membrane leads to impairment of breathing, sucking, thermoregulation and mobility. When the membrane sheds there is a risk of fluid/electrolyte imbalance and infection. Sixty per cent of babies with a collodion membrane will go on to develop an ichthyosis, most commonly lamellar ichthyosis. Babies should be admitted to a neonatal unit for monitoring and kept in a warm, moist environment.

### 144 B. Autosomal dominant

Darier's disease is inherited in an autosomal dominant manner with variable expressivity. The genetic defect is in the ATP2A2 gene on chromosome 12 that codes for a calcium ATPase. The condition presents in young adulthood with a keratotic and crusted greasy papular rash that may form malodorous plaques. The rash has a seborrhoeic distribution and is aggravated by heat, humidity and sunlight. Palmar-plantar pustules, oral lesions and nail abnormalities are also seen. Rarely segmental and acral haemorrhagic forms may be seen. Severe forms of Darier's disease may be associated with short stature and mental retardation. The skin lesions have a classical histology with acantholytic dyskeratosis, suprabasal clefting and corps ronds and grains. Treatment is with antibiotics and systemic retinoids.

### 145 A. Precocious puberty

Tuberous sclerosis is a genodermatosis inherited in an autosomal dominant fashion but up to three-quarters of cases are the result of new mutations. Mutations are seen in the TSC1 and TSC2 genes which code for the tumour suppressor proteins hamartin and tuberin. There is variation in gene penetrance and expressivity leading to a wide spectrum of disease severity.

Cutaneous features of tuberous sclerosis:
• ash leaf macules – hypopigmented patches on trunk, present from birth

- adenoma sebaceum – facial angiofibromas, present from age four
- shagreen patches – connective tissue naevi seen on the back and neck
- periungual fibromas – occur as patients get older
- skin tags, café au lait macules, poliosis
- gingival fibromas, dental enamel pits.

Other features of tuberous sclerosis:

- retinal astrocytic hamartomas (phakomas), coloboma, angiofibromas of the eyelid
- cardiac rhabdomyoma – often present at birth and shrinks
- lung cysts
- angiomyolipomas of kidney, renal cysts, renal cell carcinoma
- learning difficulties, seizures, autism, psychiatric illness
- giant cell astrocytoma, cortical tubers, sub-ependymal nodules, intracranial calcification, hydrocephalus.

In this question all the features described are seen in tuberous sclerosis except for precocious puberty which is a feature of the genodermatosis McCune-Albright syndrome.

## 146 E. Ehlers-Danlos syndrome

Café au lait macules (CALMs) are flat, round, well-circumscribed light brown patches that are present at, or soon after birth and may increase in size and number with age. Up to 30% of the population has a small number of CALMs, patients with greater than 5 CALMs should be assessed for neurofibromatosis.

Neurofibromatosis type 1 is a genodermatosis with autosomal dominant inheritance, high penetrance and variable expressivity. A mutation is seen in the NF1 gene that codes for the neurofibromin protein on chromosome 17q. Features include:

- cutaneous and plexiform neurofibromas, nerve sheath tumours
- macrocephaly, astrocytoma
- axillary and groin freckling, large congenital naevi, xanthogranulomas
- multiple CALMs
- sphenoid dysplasia, cortical thinning of long bones, kyphoscoliosis, pseudoarthrosis
- Lisch nodules in iris, optic glioma
- acromegaly, Addison's, phaeochromocytoma, precocious puberty
- sarcomas.

Neurofibromatosis type 2 is due to a mutation in the NF2 gene on chromosome 22q that codes for the cytoskeletal protein merlin.

Features include:
- bilateral acoustic neuromas
- multiple CALMs
- intracranial and spinal tumours
- neurofibromas are often absent.

Other syndromes with CALMs include:
- McCune-Albright syndrome
- Jaffe-Campanacci syndrome
- Cowden's disease
- Bloom syndrome
- piebaldism
- tuberous sclerosis
- ataxia telangiectasia
- Westerhof syndrome
- Silver Russell syndrome
- multiple endocrine neoplasia type II
- Turner's syndrome.

In this question all the syndromes mentioned feature a pathological number of café au lait macules with the exception of the skin hyperextensibility disorder Ehlers-Danlos syndrome.

## 147 B. Collagen

Ehlers-Danlos syndrome is a group of congenital disorders characterised by defects in collagen. Gene mutations may affect collagen itself or one of a number of enzymes involved in the post-translational modification of collagen. It may be inherited in an autosomal dominant or autosomal recessive fashion. The clinical features of Ehlers-Danlos are variable depending on the gene involved and type of mutation and may include:
- hyperextensible, fragile skin with poor wound healing
- molluscoid pseudotumors of the skin, bruising, Raynaud's phenomenon
- joint hypermobility and instability, congenital hip dislocation, early onset osteoarthritis
- flat feet, scoliosis, kyphosis, tethered spinal cord, carpal tunnel syndrome
- arterial rupture, aneurysms, valvular heart disease
- uterine rupture, hernias, intestinal rupture
- muscle hypotonia and weakness
- spontaneous pneumothorax

- blue sclera
- high, narrow arched palate with dental crowding.

## 148 D. Pseudoxanthoma elasticum

Pseudoxanthoma elasticum (PXE) is a genodermatosis characterised by abnormalities in the skin, eyes and cardiovascular system. Most cases are due to a mutation in the ABCC6 gene and are inherited in an autosomal recessive fashion. Other mutations and autosomal dominant inheritance have been described. In PXE there is distortion of elastic fibres and deposition of calcium in the dermis and blood vessels. Features of the disorder include:

- yellow skin with papules, cobblestoning and redundant folds of skin most prominent of the lateral neck and flexures
- defects in Bruch's membrane leading to angioid streaks and possible loss of visual acuity
- calcification of medium sized arteries leading to claudication, hypertension, myocardial infarction, stroke, retinal haemorrhage, renal artery stenosis and gastrointestinal bleeding
- strong association with Paget's disease of the bones.

In this question the patient has the typical skin signs of PXE and there is a family history of a similar skin condition associated with early myocardial infarction.

## 149 E. Dowling-Meara

Epidermolysis bullosa (EB) is a group of congenital disorders characterised by skin fragility and blistering. Defects in specific proteins lead to splits in the skin, the depth of these splits are strongly correlated with the clinical phenotype as shown in Table 8.3.

**Table 8.3** Epidermolysis bullosa according to the depth of the cutaneous split

| Type of EB | Inheritance | Split | Phenotype |
| --- | --- | --- | --- |
| EB Simplex | Autosomal dominant | Intraepidermal split | Generally mild, bullae induced by friction, worse in heat |
| Junctional EB | Autosomal recessive | Lamina-lucida split | Variable severity, mild to fatal |
| Dystrophic EB | Autosomal dominant or autosomal recessive | Sub-epidermal split | Scarring, mild to severe |

**Table 8.4** Important subtypes of EB and their clinical features

| Name | Type of EB | Clinical features |
| --- | --- | --- |
| Weber-Cockayne | EB simplex | Mild form of EB, flaccid blisters on hands and feet related to friction |
| Koebner | EB simplex | Bullae at birth, improves by adolescence, milia, some nail dystrophy |
| Dowling-Meara | EB simplex | Widespread severe bullae at birth which may be fatal, improves with age, bullae have herpetiform grouping, palmar-plantar keratoderma |
| Non-Herlitz | Junctional EB | Blisters, scarring, dystrophic nails, scarring alopecia, normal growth and lifespan |
| Herlitz | Junctional EB | Extensive skin and mucous membrane scarring bullae, paronychial inflammation, dysplastic teeth, often fatal early in life |
| Recessive | Dystrophic EB | Widespread dystrophy and scarring, nail and mucous membrane involvement, mitten deformity hands and feet, contractures, eye problems, aphonia, alopecia, skin cancer, variable degree of severity |
| Dominant | Dystrophic EB | Intermittent blistering episodes that improve with age, mild hair and nail problems, hypertrophic/atrophic scars with milia, normal lifespan |

There are no interventional treatments for EB, patients require a multidisciplinary approach to their care with input from a specialised unit. Diagnosis is normally from a skin biopsy sent to a national reference laboratory, in some families the genetic mutation is known and can be screened for. Prenatal diagnosis may be undertaken with a foetal skin biopsy or chorionic villus sampling if the mutation is known.

In this question the patient has a typical history of EB Dowling-Meara with severe blistering at birth and herpetiform blistering as a teenager.

## 150 A. Autosomal recessive

Albinism is the congenital absence of pigmentation and may affect the skin, eyes and hair and tends to be classified as ocular or oculocutaneous depending on whether the eyes, skin and hair are affected. Most cases are inherited in an autosomal recessive fashion but autosomal dominant and x-linked recessive forms are also described.

Clinical features of albinism may include:
* iris translucency, can be pink, blue or brown

- skin may be white, yellow, cream or tan colour
- hair may be white, yellow, red, cream or light brown
- photosensitivity
- increased risk of skin cancer
- nystagmus, strabismus, refractive errors, macular hypoplasia.

In albinism there is a defect in melanin synthesis that is often due to a mutation in tyrosinase, a key enzyme which catalyses the oxidation of tyrosine.

**Table 8.5** Common types of albinism and albinism 'plus' syndromes

| Disorder | Defect | Phenotype |
| --- | --- | --- |
| OCA1 | Complete lack of tyrosinase activity | White hair, white skin, pink or blue eyes |
| OCA2, OCA3, OCA4 | Reduced tyrosinase activity | Variable severity – may be near normal or like OCA1 |
| Hermansky-Pudlak syndrome | Abnormality of lysosomal function | Oculocutaneous albinism, platelet dysfunction, immunodeficiency |
| Chediak-Higashi syndrome | Lysosomal regulating defect | Immunodeficiency, bleeding defect, partial albinism |
| Griscelli syndrome | Defect in microtubule transportation | Immunodeficiency, albinism, often fatal |
| Waardenburg syndrome | – | White forelock, deafness, neural crest abnormalities, albinism |
| Tietz syndrome | Defect in the microphthalmia-associated transcription factor | Deafness, albinism |

In this question the child has oculocutaneous albinism, the commonest type of inheritance for this condition is autosomal recessive.

## 151 C. Ataxia telangiectasia

Ataxia telangiectasia is a rare congenital disorder due to a mutation in the ATM gene, it is inherited in an autosomal recessive fashion. Patients present as toddlers with cerebellar ataxia and go on to develop telangiectasia from the age of five years. Clinical features include:

- progressive cerebellar ataxia, ocular apraxia
- oculocutaneous telangiectasia

- immunodeficiency, low immunoglobulin levels, recurrent sinus and pulmonary infections
- chromosomal instability
- hypersensitivity to ionising radiation
- increased risk of malignancy especially lymphoma and leukaemia
- thymic hypoplasia.

There are no specific treatments for ataxia telangiectasia, most patients die as young adults from infection or malignancy.

Hereditary haemorrhagic telangiectasia (Osler-Weber-Rendu disease) is a rare disorder of multiple mucocutaneous and gastrointestinal telangiectasia. It is due to mutations in the HHT1 and HHT2 genes and inherited in an autosomal dominant fashion. Features include:

- characteristic mat-like telangiectasia on the skin and mucous membranes appear in adolescence and worsen with age
- involvement of the gastrointestinal tract and internal organs leads to gastrointestinal bleeding, iron deficiency anaemia, pulmonary arteriovenous fistulae, high output heart failure and persistent epistaxis.

The telangiectasia may be treated with diathermy, cautery, laser or embolisation.

**Table 8.6** Disorders of congenital/paediatric telangiectasia

| Disorder | Features |
| --- | --- |
| Angioma serpiginosum | Harmless patches of telangiectasia occur in a serpiginous or gyrate pattern on the skin in early childhood |
| Unilateral naevoid telangiectasia | Patches of telangiectasia occurring in a unilateral linear distribution, may be congenital or acquired |
| Hereditary benign telangiectasia | An autosomal dominant disorder of telangiectasia occurring on the face, trunk and arms. Similar to hereditary haemorrhagic telangiectasia but without epistaxis and visceral involvement |
| Cutis marmorata telangiectatica congenita | A congenital cutaneous syndrome of reticulated vasculature, telangiectasia, atrophic depressions and associated abnormalities |

In this question the patient has progressive ataxia and oculocutaneous telangiectasia consistent with a diagnosis of ataxia telangiectasia.

**152 E. Serum zinc level**

Acrodermatitis enteropathica is an eczematous skin rash related to zinc deficiency. It may be congenital or acquired secondary to prematurity or dietary deficiency. The congenital form is due to a mutation in a transmembrane zinc uptake protein and is inherited in an autosomal recessive fashion. Features include:

- a sharply demarcated, eroded, crusty eczematous rash in a perioral and perianal distribution, occasionally the rash may become bullous, eroded or pustular
- diarrhoea
- paronychia
- alopecia
- growth failure
- anaemia
- poor wound healing
- mental retardation
- death.

It often presents in children at the time of weaning and can be diagnosed by a reduced serum zinc level. Treatment is with zinc supplementation.

In this question a young child is presenting with treatment resistant eczema in a perioral and perianal distribution and mild alopecia. This picture is suspicious of acrodermatitis enteropathica and a serum zinc level should be measured. It is unlikely that any form of allergy testing would be helpful in a child of this age.

**153 B. Irritant contact dermatitis**

Napkin (diaper) dermatitis is a common rash seen in nappy wearing children and is characterised by patches of erythema and scaling that spare the groin folds. It is due to an irritant contact dermatitis resulting from prolonged exposure of the skin to urine and stool. In breastfed babies the stool has a lower pH and lower enzyme activity resulting in a lower incidence of napkin dermatitis. It is most common in children of 6–12 months of age as they start to wean and the composition of the stool changes. Secondary bacterial or fungal infection may complicate napkin dermatitis with the rash spreading to the groin folds and satellite lesions appearing around the border. Treatment of napkin dermatitis involves barrier creams, regular nappy changes and mild topical steroids.

**Table 8.7** Dermatoses affecting the nappy area

| Disorder | Features |
|---|---|
| Psoriasis | Scattered beefy red papules which may coalesce into well defined plaques, often lacks scale, look for other skin/nail signs of psoriasis or a family history |
| Primary candidiasis | Erythema with satellite pustules, may be sharply demarcated with a raised edge, involves groin folds, often follows systemic antibiotics |
| Acrodermatitis enteropathica | Treatment resistant eczematous looking rash, may blister or become crusty, look for perioral involvement, *see* question 152 |
| Granuloma gluteale infantum | Red-purple granulomatous nodules, a foreign body reaction to talc or barrier preparations, benign and self limiting |
| Langerhans cell histiocytosis | Erythema and scale, progresses to purpuric nodules, extremely rare and may be serious, *see* question 158 |

In this question the child has an irritated, erythematous rash in the nappy area and the history of a soiled nappy and unkempt child hints towards neglect or a parent who is having difficulty coping. The lack of satellite lesions and sparing of the groin folds is clinically typical of napkin dermatitis, an irritant contact dermatitis to urine and stool.

## 154 B. Hyperhidrosis
Ectodermal dysplasias are a collection of over 150 syndromes caused by defects in the ectodermal structures. They are due to mutations in a number of different genes and may arise de novo or be inherited in a recessive, dominant or x-linked fashion. Features include:
- hair that may be fragile, sparse, curly or hypopigmented with poor or no growth
- dystrophic nails which may be thickened, discoloured and brittle, paronychia is common
- hypo and hyperpigmentation of the skin, palmoplantar keratoderma, xerosis, infections
- hypohidrosis
- absent, peg-shaped or pointed teeth, enamel defects
- abnormal facies with frontal bossing, pronounced chin and a broad nose
- eye and ear abnormalities
- recurrent respiratory tract infections, chronic nasal/sinus infections
- cleft palate/lip

- missing fingers or toes
- poor breast development.

There is no specific treatment for ectodermal dysplasia and patients should be managed in a multi-disciplinary fashion with early input from dentists.

In this question hyperhidrosis is not a commonly seen feature of ectodermal dysplasia. Hypohidrosis is well described as are cleft palate, pigmentary change, dental abnormalities and dystrophic nails.

## 155 E. Bland emollients

Gianotti-Crosti syndrome is also known as papular acrodermatitis of childhood and is a rare eruption that often follows an upper respiratory tract infection and can be associated with mild systemic upset. It affects children of any age with an equal sex distribution. A previous epidemic in Japan was associated with the hepatitis B surface antigen. The rash consists of multiple small monomorphous lichenoid papules that may be skin coloured or red. It is non-itchy, symmetrical and affects the face, extremities, buttocks, palms and soles. It may be associated with a low grade fever, lymphadenopathy and hepatosplenomegaly. The rash is self-limiting and normally settles in 2–8 weeks. Treatment is with emollients, topical steroids may exacerbate the condition.

In this question the patient has a history and examination typical of Gianotti-Crosti syndrome, the rash is self limiting and treatment is with emollients.

## 156 E. Striae

Marfan's syndrome is a congenital disorder of connective tissue. A mutation is seen in the FBN1 gene which codes for the fibrillin-1 protein. The mutation either arises de novo or is inherited in an autosomal dominant fashion. Features include:

- tall stature with long slender limbs and arachnodactyly, scoliosis, pectus excavatum, pectus carinatum, joint hyperextensibility, high thin arched palate, flat feet, hammer toes, thin wrists, speech defects, early osteoarthritis
- striae, elastosis perforans serpiginosa, thin slightly hyperextensible skin
- mitral and aortic valve prolapse, aortic regurgitation, aortic aneurysm, aortic dissection
- upwards lens dislocation, astigmatism, retinal detachment, glaucoma

- spontaneous pneumothorax
- dural ectasia, dysautonomia.

In this question striae are a well recognised cutaneous feature of Marfan's syndrome. Downwards (inferonasal) dislocation of the lens is a typical feature of homocystinuria, in Marfan's syndrome lens dislocation is superior (superotemporal).

## 157 C. Mast cells circulating in peripheral blood

Mastocytosis is an abnormal collection of mast cells in the skin or internal organs. Fifty per cent of mastocytosis cases occur in children where it has a good prognosis.

**Table 8.8** Subtypes of mastocytosis

| Type of Mastocytosis | Description |
| --- | --- |
| Solitary mastocytoma | A single red-brown lesion that may be a macule or papule and measure from a few mm to several cm in size. It may be present at birth or appear in infancy. When stroked it becomes urticated and possibly bullous (Darier's sign). Other causes of degranulation include exercise, hot baths and histamine releasing drugs (alcohol, codeine, dextran). Systemic disease is not seen and it has an excellent prognosis |
| Urticaria pigmentosa | Multiple red-brown lesions in early childhood, it is most commonly seen on the trunk. Individual lesions show Darier's sign. If multiple lesions degranulate the patient may develop systemic symptoms such as flush, hypotension, headache, diarrhoea, wheezing and syncope. Systemic disease is rare and the lesions tend to resolve as children enter adolescence |
| Diffuse cutaneous mastocytosis | Rare, this may be present from birth or arise before the age of three years. The skin may look normal or have red-brown macules and plaques that become confluent. When degranulated the skin develops a boggy, leathery texture with vesicles. Systemic involvement may occur in the childhood form and is common in adult disease |
| Systemic mastocytosis | Rarely seen in paediatric disease. Patients may have skeletal lesions, bone marrow infiltration, splenomegaly, lymphadenopathy and gastrointestinal involvement. Serum mast cell tryptase level is often raised |
| Mast cell leukaemia | The presence of mast cells in the peripheral blood is an indicator of poor prognosis. Mast cell leukaemia is defined as when greater than 10% of peripheral blood nucleated cells are mast cells. Prognosis is poor with few patients surviving more than a year from diagnosis |

Treatment is not required for most patients and they only need to avoid precipitants of mast cell degranulation. When treatment is needed it is aimed at symptom relief with antihistamines, sodium cromoglycate, cimetidine and PUVA. Aggressive forms of mastocytosis are treated with interferon-alpha, cladribine and imantinib mesylate.

In this question mast cells circulating in the blood carries the worst prognosis as this is associated with mast cell leukaemia. Mast cells in the bone marrow and a raised serum mast cell tryptase level are associated with systemic mastocytosis. The number of skin lesions and whether they blister is not related to overall prognosis.

## 158 A. Hepatosplenomegaly

Langerhans cell histiocytosis (LCH) is a rare disease that results from a clonal proliferation of Langerhans cells. It has previously been called Hans-Schüller-Christian disease, Letterer-Siwe disease and histiocytosis X. The clonal Langerhans cells combine with lymphocytes, eosinophils and histiocytes to form the multinucleated giant cells and granulomas typical of LCH.

**Table 8.9** Subtypes of Langerhans cell histiocytosis

| Type of LCH | Age affected | Prognosis | Features |
|---|---|---|---|
| Unifocal LCH (Eosinophilic granuloma) | Over 6 years | Good | Slowly progressive single lesion in bone, skin or soft tissues. Often an osteolytic lesion in a long or flat bone, it may also present as an ulcer, otitis media (mastoid lesion) or tooth disruption (jaw lesion). Treated with curettage or low dose radiotherapy. 10% progress to multifocal disease |
| Multifocal unisystem LCH | 3–6 years | Moderate | Classical triad of diabetes insipidus (pituitary involvement), exopthalmos and lytic bone lesions. It may also present with a seborrhoeic dermatitis-like rash, ulceration, bone pain and chronic cough. Treated with radiotherapy and chemotherapy. Spontaneous remission is possible, lung involvement is a poor sign |

*continued*

**Table 8.9** *continued*

| Multifocal multisystem LCH (Malignant Letterer-Siwe disease) | Less 3 years | Poor | Rapidly progressive multisystem disease. Patients may be systemically unwell with a generalised skin eruption, multiple LCH lesions, anaemia, hepatosplenomegaly, lymphadenopathy and lung involvement. Treatment is with immunosuppressives and chemotherapy. It is often fulminant and fatal |

In this question hepatosplenomegaly is not typical of multifocal unisystem Langerhans cell histiocytosis, it is more typical of multifocal multisystem (Letterer-Siwe) disease.

### 159 E. Aplasia cutis

Aplasia Cutis is a congenital defect of the skin, usually the scalp, where there is localised loss of tissue. There is variation in the size and depth of skin loss which may be epidermal, dermal or subcutaneous. The defect presents as a midline ulcer at birth that heals with scarring. Surgical correction may be needed as the patch of scarring alopecia is permanent. Aplasia cutis is only rarely associated with other developmental abnormalities.

The vernix caseosa is an adherent white-grey greasy membrane that protects the skin in utero. It may be present at birth and is slowly shed over a few weeks and its presence is physiological and not associated with any disorders. It should be differentiated from the thicker, more rigid membrane of a collodion baby (*see* question 143).

Cutis marmorata is seen as reticulated mottling of the skin in newborns. It appears in the cold and resolves on warming. Treatment is not needed and the mottling resolves by 1 month of age. It should not be confused with the vascular disorder cutis marmorata telangiectasia congenita (*see* question 151).

Milia are 1–2 mm superficial epidermoid cysts that are commonly seen on the faces of newborn babies and they resolve within a few weeks. Rarely milia may be associated with disorders such as epidermolysis bullosa and hereditary trichodysplasia.

Miliaria crystalline are superficial pinpoint vesicles seen in the intertriginous areas. They are due to the blockage of sweat ducts and are commonly seen in newborns. Cooling of the baby leads to rapid resolution of the lesions. Miliaria rubra are a similar phenomenon except the vesicles are erythematous. Both of the rashes are related to physiologically immature adnexal structures and are not associated with any pathological disorders.

In this question aplasia cutis is pathological, the other rashes are physiological.

## 160 C. Up to 5 days

Erythema toxicum neonatorum is a benign, transient rash that is commonly seen in newborn babies. It presents between 24–48 hours of age and clears over 5 days, by 2 weeks of age the rash has always resolved. It presents as 2–3 cm diameter blotchy erythematous macules with central vesicles, papules or pustules. It does not require treatment.

Transient neonatal pustular melanosis is a similar benign self limiting condition of newborns. It is more commonly seen in Afro-Caribbean babies, presenting with blotchy erythema and pustules. When the pustules heal hyperpigmentation is left behind that fades over 3–6 months. The rash occurs with an analogous timescale to erythema toxicum neonatorum and follows a similar benign, self-resolving course.

In this question the patient has features typical of erythema toxicum neonatorum, it should resolve in 4–5 days.

## 161 D. Congenital cytomegalovirus infection

Blueberry muffin babies present with a widespread rash of blue-red papules and nodules at birth. The rash is due to congenital infection in utero.

**Table 8.10** Causes of a blueberry muffin baby

| Disease | Additional features |
| --- | --- |
| Toxoplasmosis | Hepatosplenomegaly, lymphadenopathy, hydrocephalus, retinitis and seizures. Prognosis is poor |
| Herpes zoster | Scarring, limb contractures, encephalitis, malformed limbs, growth retardation |
| Human immunodeficiency virus | Babies may have opportunistic infections and hepatosplenomegaly |
| Cytomegalovirus | May be severe with deafness, mental retardation and seizures |
| Rubella | Mental retardation, deafness, microcephaly, cataracts, hepatosplenomegaly, pneumonitis, myocarditis, encephalitis, retinopathy |

Neonatal herpes simplex infection occurs during delivery with direct spread from vaginal lesions. Up to 70% of patients have no skin lesions, when lesions do occur they are typically papules that progress to grouped vesicles. The infection may be limited to the skin, involve the central nervous system or can be disseminated. Untreated disseminated infection has a mortality of over 80%.

Congenital syphilis occurs when the mother has active secondary or tertiary syphilis. Half of pregnancies result in miscarriage. Of the babies who survive 10% die in infancy due to pulmonary haemorrhage. Features include:

- deafness
- Hutchinson's teeth, mulberry molars
- interstitial keratitis
- frontal bossing, sabre shins, saddle nose
- poorly developed muscles
- hepatosplenomegaly, anaemia, jaundice, lymphadenopathy
- petechiae, bullous lesions on palms and soles, maculopapular or papulosquamous lesions on the body, mucous membrane patches, anogenital plaques.

In this question the child is presenting with a blueberry muffin appearance, of the possible answers congenital cytomegalovirus infection is the most likely cause.

## 162 A. Calcium

Subcutaneous fat necrosis of the newborn is a rare condition seen in babies of 2–3 weeks of age. It presents with one or more erythematous subcutaneous nodules that may coalesce into plaques. It is often precipitated by cold and seen on the trunk, arms, buttocks, thighs and cheeks. Rarely the skin may ulcerate and necrotic fat may exude. It can be associated with significant hypercalcaemia that may require treatment. The condition is self limiting and resolves over a few months.

In this question it is important to check a serum calcium level and treat any underlying hypercalcaemia.

# Chapter 9
# Photodermatology

## QUESTIONS

**163** What colour does tinea versicolor fluoresce with Wood's light:

A   does not fluoresce
B   green
C   yellow-golden
D   blue
E   red.

**164** Thirty minutes after exposure to sunlight a patient with Fitzpatrick type II skin develops visible darkening of the skin. What is the biological mechanism that has led to this:

A   increased production of melanin
B   oxidation of melanin polymer and rearrangement of melanosomes
C   increased production and rearrangement of melanosomes
D   oxidation of melanin by photo-induced free radicals
E   formation of melanin polymers by UVA induced photosynthesis.

**165** You review a patient with chronic plaque psoriasis and decide to treat them with narrow band UVB phototherapy. What regime of treatment would be appropriate:

A   7 times per week
B   5 times per week
C   once a week
D   once every 2 weeks
E   3 times a week.

**166** A 21-year-old woman presents with a non-specific pruritic rash in a photo-distribution. She says that the rash occurs every spring and always settles by mid-summer. The patient wishes to know if any treatment is available to stop the rash occurring. What would you recommend:

A  prednisolone 30 mg once daily for 5 days
B  hydroxychloroquine
C  ciclosporin 3 mg/kg during the summer months
D  venesection of 3 units of blood
E  a short course of UVB phototherapy.

**167** Which of the following histories is typical for actinic prurigo:

A  itchy eczematous rash worse in spring, clears in the summer
B  urticated itchy rash worse in spring, clears in the summer
C  papular non-itchy rash worse in spring, clears in winter
D  itchy eczematous rash worse in summer, clears in winter
E  urticated itchy rash worse in summer, clears in winter.

**168** A 33-year-old man presents with a troublesome rash related to sun exposure. Within a few minutes of exposure to the sun his skin develops itchy wheals that fade over a few hours. Which of the following would be an appropriate treatment for his condition:

A  antihistamines
B  methotrexate
C  thalidomide
D  aspirin
E  hydroxychloroquine.

**169** Which of the following is a well recognised cause of pellagra:

A  hyperthyroidism
B  dapsone therapy
C  carcinoid syndrome
D  renal failure
E  porphyria cutanea tarda.

**170** You review a young child with photodamaged skin, eye problems and developmental delay. You suspect a diagnosis of xeroderma pigmentosum (XP). What mode of inheritance do most cases of XP exhibit:

A   autosomal dominant
B   autosomal recessive
C   x-linked recessive
D   x-linked dominant
E   mitochondrial.

**171** You are asked to review a young boy with photosensitivity. You are struck by the prominent poikiloderma on his face and suspect Rothmund-Thomson syndrome. A mutation in what gene is responsible for this condition:

A   TGM1
B   DHCR7
C   BLM
D   TTDN1
E   RecQL4.

**172** Which of the following photosensitive disorders can be treated with a high cholesterol diet:

A   Bloom's syndrome
B   Smith-Lemi-Opitz syndrome
C   xeroderma pigmentosum
D   chronic actinic dermatitis
E   Kindler syndrome.

**173** A middle-aged male patient presents with bullae and scarring on his scalp and the dorsum of his hands. You suspect that he has active porphyria cutanea tarda. What is the probability that his serum sample will have raised porphyrin levels:

A   100%
B   80%
C   50%
D   10%
E   0%.

**174** You review a 36-year-old South African patient who has been admitted to hospital with an acute attack of variegate porphyria. Which of the following drugs should she avoid whilst in hospital:

A   penicillin
B   spironolactone
C   oral contraceptive medications
D   hydroxychloroquine
E   atenolol.

**175** Which of the following is a clinical feature of erythropoietic protoporphyria:

A   gallstones
B   delayed photo-related urticaria
C   renal failure
D   cardiac failure
E   skin fragility.

## ANSWERS

### 163 C. Yellow-golden

Wood's light is a long wave ultraviolet A lamp with a nickel oxide filter. It can be used to aid in the diagnosis of a number of dermatological conditions as shown in Table 9.1.

**Table 9.1** Conditions that fluoresce with Wood's light

| Condition | Fluorescence under Wood's light |
|-----------|--------------------------------|
| Tinea versicolor | Hypopigmented macules fluoresce yellow-golden |
| Trichophyton schoenleinii tinea capitis | Infected hair fluoresces pale green |
| Microsporum audouinii tinea capitis | Infected hair fluoresces bright green |
| Microsporum canis tinea capitis | Infected hair fluoresces bright green |
| Microsporum distortum, gypseum, and nanum | May fluoresce |
| Pseudomonas aeruginosa | Fluoresces green-blue |
| Erythrasma | Corynebacterium fluoresce coral red |
| Porphyria | Urine fluoresces pink-orange |
| Vitiligo, albinism | Depigmentation is more pronounced |
| Tuberous sclerosis | Ash-leaf-macules fluoresce white |
| Ethylene glycol poisoning | Fluoresces urine |

In this question tinea versicolor fluoresces yellow-golden.

### 164 B. Oxidation of melanin polymer and rearrangement of melanosomes

This patient has type II skin on the Fitzpatrick scale, a numerical classification of skin colour. The Fitzpatrick scale is a useful tool for predicting how likely a patient is to burn after exposure to ultraviolet (UV) light.

**Table 9.2** The Fitzpatrick scale of skin pigmentation

| Fitzpatrick type | Patient complexion | Likelihood of burning after UV exposure |
|------------------|--------------------|----------------------------------------|
| Type I | Fair white skin, red hair, blue or green eyes, freckles | Always burns, never tans |

*continued*

**Table 9.2** *continued*

| Type II | Fair white skin, blonde hair, blue or green eyes | Usually burns, rarely tans |
|---------|--------------------------------------------------|----------------------------|
| Type III | Darker white skin, any hair or eye colour | Sometimes burns, gradually tans |
| Type IV | Olive/Mediterranean skin, dark hair and eyes | Rarely burns, tans easily |
| Type V | Dark brown skin, dark hair and eyes | Very rarely burns, tans very easily |
| Type VI | Black skin | Never burns, tans very easily |

After exposure to UVA radiation, patients develop immediate pigment darkening. This is the result of oxidation of melanin polymers and rearrangement of melanosomes leading to darkening of the skin which occurs within minutes and lasts less than a day. After exposure to erythema doses of UVB a delayed tan occurs due to increased production of melanin, this occurs within a few days and lasts for several weeks.

**Table 9.3** Wavelengths of the visible and ultraviolet spectrum

| Name | Wavelength |
|------|-----------|
| Visible light | 400 (violet)–700 nm (red) |
| UVA | 320–400 nm |
| UVB | 280–320 nm |
| UVC | 100–280 nm |

In this question the patient has developed immediate pigment darkening a few minutes after exposure to UVA radiation; this is due to the oxidation of melanin polymers and rearrangement of melanosomes.

### 165 E. 3 times a week

Phototherapy is the use of UV radiation to treat skin disorders. Four main types of phototherapy are used in dermatology practice as shown in Table 9.4.

**Table 9.4** Types of phototherapy

| Therapy | Description | Frequency of treatment |
|---|---|---|
| Broad band UVB | UVB light source of 290–320 nm | 2–5 times a week |
| Narrow band UVB | UVB light source of 311 nm (TL-01) | 2–3 times a week |
| PUVA | Psoralen and a UVA light source | 2 times a week |
| RePUVA | Systemic retinoid and psoralen and a UVA light source | 2 times a week |

UVB phototherapy is most commonly used for psoriasis, eczema and pruritus although there are a number of other indications. Recently there has been a trend towards using narrow band UVB rather than broad band as it clears psoriasis more efficiently with reduced erythema and reduced carcinogenicity. Prior to treatment with UVB a patient's skin type is assessed by establishing the minimal erythema dose (MED), once this has been established a treatment regime can be initiated. The commonest short term side affect is a sunburn-like response, long term there is a risk of photoageing and skin cancer.

For information on PUVA *see* question 191. RePUVA is the combination of a systemic retinoid and PUVA, it is more effective than PUVA with psoriasis clearing quicker with lower doses of UVA radiation.

Advantages of UVB phototherapy over PUVA:
- no photosensitising agent is needed
- eye protection is not needed after treatment (systemic psoralen)
- less side effects
- safe in pregnancy and safer in young patients
- shorter irradiation time.

Advantages of PUVA phototherapy over UVB:
- less frequent treatments
- more effective
- often works in UVB resistant dermatoses.

In this question the patient has been booked for narrow band UVB phototherapy, this is normally given three times a week.

## 166 E. A short course of UVB phototherapy

Polymorphic light eruption (PLE) is the most frequently seen acquired photosensitivity disorder. Typically it presents in young women with familial clustering. The rash has a variable morphology, most commonly papular or eczematous, is pruritic and occurs in a photo-distribution. It presents in the spring with a 6 hour to 3 day latency and lasts up to 2 weeks. By mid-summer the skin has become hardened to UV radiation and the rash settles. In most cases PLE lasts a few years and settles spontaneously.

In this question the patient has a history typical of PLE. To prevent the rash occurring the patient can be 'hardened' with a short course of UVB or PUVA phototherapy. Prednisolone is used to treat acute attacks of PLE, not prevent them. Immunosuppression, venesection and hydroxychloroquine have no role in the treatment of PLE.

It is important that true photosensitive dermatoses such as PLE are distinguished from photoaggravated dermatoses. Conditions such as psoriasis are often responsive to UV light, but in some patients UV can cause worsening of the disease.

Disorders with potential for photoaggravation:
- lupus, dermatomyositis
- eczema, psoriasis, PRP, lichen planus
- acne, rosacea, perioral dermatitis
- pemphigoid, pemphigus, linear IgA disease
- Hailey-Hailey, Darier's disease
- HZV, HSV, viral exanthems
- melasma, vitiligo
- Jessner's lymphocytic infiltrate, lymphocytoma cutis.

**167 D. Itchy eczematous rash worse in summer, clears in winter**
Actinic prurigo (Hutchinson's summer prurigo) is a rare acquired photosensitivity disorder that often presents in young adults or children. It is more common in Native Americans, females, those with a family history and there is a strong association with HLA DR4 DRB1*0407. Patients present with an itchy eczematous rash on sun exposed sites during the summer that clears during the winter, cheilitis of the lips may also occur. Patients are exceedingly sensitive to the whole UV spectrum including visible light and often covered sites are affected due to penetration of UV radiation. The prognosis is uncertain but in many cases it settles spontaneously over a number of years. Treatment includes photoprotection, topical steroids, UVB/ PUVA desensitisation, ciclosporin and thalidomide.

Hydroa vacciniforme is another rare acquired photosensitivity disorder that often presents in children. It is more common in fair skinned individuals and can show familial clustering. Patients are sensitive to UVA radiation which leads to papulovesicles and umbilicated vesicles in sun exposed sites. These lesions heal with crateriform scars and have a predilection for the face. It tends to resolve spontaneously after 2–5 years but may leave severe scarring. Treatment is with rigorous photoprotection, topical steroids, hydroxychloroquine, azathioprine and ciclosporin.

## 168 A. Antihistamines
Solar urticaria is rare accounting for less than 1% of all urticarias. It is seen in young adults and has a slight female predominance. Urticaria occurs within minutes of sun exposure and fades over a few hours. Patients may be sensitive to different wavelengths of UV radiation with UVA and visible light being the commonest. The condition is often chronic and may last many years. Treatment is with photoprotection, antihistamines and plasmapheresis.

In this question the patient has a history typical of solar urticaria and first line treatment with photoprotection and antihistamines would be appropriate.

Chronic actinic dermatitis (CAD) is another rare acquired photosensitive disorder. It is most commonly seen in elderly men who are exceedingly sensitive to UVA, UVB and the visible spectrum. Patients present with severe confluent eczema of sun exposed sites with striking cut off at the collars and cuffs. The rash is constant during the summer and fades during the winter. CAD may follow a photosensitive drug reaction and patients frequently show positive type IV allergic reactions. Treatment is with photoprotection, topical steroids, ciclosporin and azathioprine. The disorder often settles spontaneously after a few years.

## 169 C. Carcinoid syndrome
Pellagra is due to deficiency of niacin (nicotinic acid, vitamin B3), tryptophan or leucine. Patients presents with 'the four Ds':
- diarrhoea
- dermatitis
- dementia
- death.

Skin lesions may be erythematous, pigmented or indurated and are seen on sun exposed sites, cheilitis is also common. Treatment is with 300 mg/day oral niacin supplements and a healthy diet.

Causes include:

- low protein diet (e.g. maize rich diet)
- Hartnup disease
- alcoholism
- malabsorption
- liver failure
- carcinoid syndrome
- isoniazid.

In this question the well recognised cause is carcinoid syndrome where altered protein metabolism leads to a relative tryptophan deficiency.

Hartnup disease is a rare autosomal recessive disorder of neutral amino-acid transport. Patients present aged 3–9 years with a pellagra-like photosensitive rash, cerebellar ataxia, mental retardation, oedema and a fatty liver. The prognosis is good, patients can be treated with nicotinic acid supplements and a high protein diet.

## 170 B. Autosomal recessive

Xeroderma pigmentosum (XP) is a very rare disorder of congenital photosensitivity. Eighty per cent of patients have a defect in DNA excision repair (classical XP), 20% have a defect in daughter strand repair (XP variant). In answer to the question, both forms are inherited in an autosomal recessive manner and have an equal sex distribution. Patients often present in childhood after suffering an exaggerated sunburn response. As patients get older they develop severe photodamage and multiple skin cancers. Eye and neurological complications are frequently seen. The gold standard for diagnosis is UV irradiated skin fibroblast culture; photoprovocation and genetic testing are helpful in some cases. Treatment is with rigorous photoprotection, cancer surveillance and psychological support.

Trichothiodystrophy is another very rare autosomal recessive disorder of congenital photosensitivity. Up to 50% of patients have defective nucleotide excision repair showing overlap with XP. The degree of photosensitivity is variable and there is no increased risk of skin cancer. Other features include chronic ichthyosis, sparse brittle hair, typical facies, short stature, mental retardation, erythroderma, eczema, multiple infections, cataracts, dental caries and hypoplastic nails. Diagnosis is made with UV irradiated skin fibroblast culture, monochromator testing is normal.

Cockayne syndrome is a congenital disorder that may also overlap with XP showing photosensitivity. It has autosomal recessive inheritance with significant variation in phenotypic severity. Patients often present a few hours after sun exposure when they develop a scaly, erythematous rash. Over time the rash may lead to pigmentation and scarring although there is no increased risk of skin cancer. Other features include short stature, mental retardation, large hands, feet and ears, eye problems and deafness. The photosensitivity resolves with age but prognosis is very poor with death before the age of 20 from progressive neurological demyelination.

## 171 E. RecQL4

Rothmund-Thomson syndrome is a rare autosomal recessive congenital photosensitivity syndrome related to a DNA helicase mutation. It is characterised by the development of prominent poikiloderma within the first year of life. Other features include photosensitivity, warty hyperkeratosis, cataracts, short stature, skeletal dysplasia and an increased risk of Bowen's disease and osteosarcoma.

Kindler syndrome is another rare autosomal recessive congenital photosensitivity syndrome with poikiloderma. Mutations in the Kind-1 gene lead to a defect in actin binding in the extracellular matrix. Patients develop blistering and skin fragility in infancy that is often indistinguishable from epidermolysis bullosa. Other features include progressive and generalised poikiloderma, diffuse cutaneous atrophy, palmar hyperkeratosis, gingivitis, urethral, oesophageal and anal stenosis.

In this question the gene responsible for Rothmund-Thomson syndrome is RecQL4. TGM1 gene mutations are seen in lamellar ichthyosis, DHCR7 mutations are seen in Smith-Lemi-Opitz syndrome, BLM mutations are seen in Bloom's syndrome and TTDN1 mutations are seen in trichothiodystrophy.

## 172 B. Smith-Lemi-Opitz syndrome

Smith-Lemi-Opitz syndrome is an autosomal recessive congenital disorder of cholesterol synthesis. Two-thirds of patients have photosensitivity with an exaggerated sunburn response to UVA. Other features include mental retardation, ambiguous genitalia, dysmorphic facies, failure to thrive, cleft palate, congenital heart disease and polydactyly. Treatment includes photoprotection and a high cholesterol diet.

Bloom's syndrome is another autosomal recessive congenital photosensitivity disorder. It is rare and most commonly seen in Ashkenazi Jews. Features include growth retardation, typical facies, telangiectasia and erythema of sun exposed skin, hyper and hypo-pigmentation and significant immunodeficiency. There is a very high risk of malignancy especially leukaemia, gastrointestinal, breast and skin cancer. A mutation is seen in the BLM gene that has a role in DNA replication forks.

## 173 A. 100%

Porphyrias are disorders of haem synthesis. In cutaneous porphyrias unstable intermediates in the haem pathway build up in the skin where they undergo UV induced degradation into free radicals that damage surrounding cells. In this question the patient has an active skin porphyria and therefore must have raised serum porphyrins.

Porphyria cutanea tarda (PCT) is the commonest cutaneous porphyria and occurs with a slight male predominance in middle-aged adults. Most cases are acquired, 20% are congenital when it is inherited in an autosomal dominant fashion. Patients have a defect in uroporphyrinogen decarboxylase leading to an accumulation of porphyrins in the liver that spill over into the serum and are activated by UV in the skin. Features include photodistributed bullae, scarring, slow healing erosions and milia. Hypertrichosis, pigmentary change, scarring alopecia, onycholysis and hepatocellular carcinoma are also seen.

Predisposing factors include:
- alcohol
- oestrogens
- hepatitis infection
- HIV infection
- haemochromatosis.

Treatment is with photoprotection, avoidance of precipitants, venesection and hydroxychloroquine. Patients need regular follow up due to the risk of hepatocellular carcinoma.

## 174 C. Oral contraceptive medications

Variegate porphyria is a rare porphyria with autosomal dominant inheritance and variable penetrance. There is a cluster of cases in South Africa. A defect is seen in the enzyme protoporphyrinogen oxidase leading to an accumulation of protoporphyrin IX. Most patients are asymptomatic, those with active disease present with the cutaneous features of PCT and acute attacks of confusion, abdominal pain, seizures and psychosis. Patients with cutaneous signs have raised serum porphyrins and those having acute attacks have raised urine porphyrins.

Precipitants of acute attacks include:

- infection
- starvation
- stress
- pregnancy
- menstruation
- alcohol, cannabis, barbiturates, anticonvulsants and progesterones.

Treatment includes photoprotection and avoiding precipitants. Acute attacks are treated with analgesia and hemantin. In this question the patient should avoid the oral contraceptive pill which contains progesterone, a known precipitant of variegate porphyria attacks.

## 175 A. Gallstones

Erythropoietic protoporphyria (EPP) is due to impaired activity of the enzyme ferrochelatase. This results in accumulation of its substrate protoporphyrin. Protoporphyrins in the skin are excited by light causing local photoxidative damage and symptoms such as immediate tingling, itching, erythema and purpura. Protoporphyrins also accumulate in the liver causing hepatic damage and are excreted in the bile predisposing to gallstones. EPP usually presents in children and has an equal sex distribution, both autosomal dominant and autosomal recessive inheritance have been reported. With time patients develop pitted scars and thickened skin on the cheeks, nose and dorsum of the hand. Treatment is with photoprotection, beta-carotene, afamelanotide, cysteine and cholestyramine. In the majority of patients the cutaneous features are mild, only a small number of patients develop significant liver disease.

In this question gallstones are a clinical feature of erythropoietic protoporphyria, the others are not.

# Chapter 10

# Dermatopharmacology

## QUESTIONS

**176** You review a 37-year-old patient with longstanding psoriasis. He has had a recent flare of his disease despite optimum topical therapies and you advise him to start methotrexate. Which of the following potential side effects are you least likely to warn the patient about:

A  hepatotoxicity
B  photosensitivity
C  pancytopenia
D  irreversible oligozoospermia
E  nausea.

**177** A 64-year-old man is under your care with longstanding psoriasis. He has taken low dose weekly methotrexate for a number a years as his primary treatment. On his most recent blood tests his Pro-collagen III NP level was 6.8, all previous results were in the normal range (1.7–4.2). What is the most appropriate course of action:

A  stop the methotrexate immediately and organise for a liver biopsy
B  stop the methotrexate immediately and monitor liver function enzymes for the next 12 months
C  reduce the dose of methotrexate and organise for a liver biopsy
D  continue with the same dose of methotrexate and repeat the test in three months
E  continue with the same dose of methotrexate and refer to a hepatologist.

**178** You review a 59-year-old woman with moderate psoriasis. Previously treatment with methotrexate, acitretin and ciclosporin has failed. You started her on hydroxycarbamide 500mg once daily four weeks ago. There is a small improvement in her psoriasis but her blood tests are now abnormal:

|  | Prior to starting therapy | Current | Normal range |
|---|---|---|---|
| HB | 11.9 | 10.3 | 11.5 to 16.5 g/dl |
| MCV | 88 | 118 | 76 to 100 fL |
| PLT | 212 | 160 | 150 to 450 x10⁹/L |
| WCC | 6.8 | 5.2 | 4 to 11 x10⁹/L |

What is the most appropriate course of action:

A   stop the hydroxycarbamide, organise for a blood transfusion
B   stop the hydroxycarbamide and monitor
C   continue with the same dose of hydroxycarbamide
D   decrease the dose of hydroxycarbamide to 250 mg once daily
E   increase the dose of hydroxycarbamide to 500 mg twice daily.

**179** You plan to start a 100 kg man on azathioprine for treatment resistant bullous pemphigoid. He has no other medical problems and baseline haematology and biochemistry tests are normal. His thiopurine s-methyltransferase (TMPT) level is reported as more than 34 U. What is would be the maximum dose safe dose of azathioprine to give this patient:

A   500 mg per day
B   250 mg per day
C   150 mg per day
D   50 mg per day
E   none.

**180** You review a 15-year-old boy with severe cystic acne who was started on isotretinoin 30 mg/day (0.5 mg/kg) three weeks ago. He feels unwell in himself with a fever, bone pain and a number of eruptive pyogenic granulomas are seen on the skin. What is the appropriate course of action:

A   continue isotretinoin and add in prednisolone 40 mg/day
B   increase isotretinoin to 1 mg/kg/day
C   stop isotretinoin
D   stop isotretinoin and start prednisolone 40 mg/kg/day
E   stop isotretinoin and start dapsone.

**181** A 27-year-old nurse with severe eczema requests for a short term improvement of her eczema over her upcoming wedding and honeymoon celebrations. After discussion and counselling it is decided to start her on ciclosporin. Her baseline blood pressure was mildly raised at 140/90. Which of the following medications is least likely to interact with ciclosporin:

A   ramipril
B   spironolactone
C   propranolol
D   diltiazem
E   verapamil.

**182** You review a young man with biopsy proven dermatitis herpetiformis. Despite potent topical steroids and a gluten free diet he is still troubled by the rash and is started on dapsone. He presents two weeks later with shortness of breath, headache, fatigue and central cyanosis. You take an arterial blood sample and note chocolate-brown discolouration of the blood. Analysis reveals a methaemoglobin level of 40%. What treatment is appropriate:

A   urgent blood transfusion
B   no treatment is indicated
C   reduce the dose of dapsone
D   amyl nitrate infusion
E   intravenous methylene blue and oxygen.

**183** When reviewing a patient with discoid lupus you discuss the option of using an anti-malarial treatment. The patient asks why she cannot combine hydroxychloroquine and mepacrine therapy. Which reason do you give:

A  ocular toxicity
B  heptotoxicity
C  haemolysis
D  hypopigmentation
E  may precipitate a pustular psoriasis.

**184** You review a patient with treatment resistant pemphigus vulgaris and start them on mycophenolate mofetil. What is the most likely side effect they may suffer from:

A  renal failure
B  gastrointestinal upset
C  anaemia
D  thrombophlebitis
E  progressive multifocal leukoencephalopathy.

**185** You are discussing possible treatment options for a female patient with discoid lupus. The patient has recently read an article on the internet about an American who had a miraculous recovery when they took thalidomide. She is keen to try the medication; she is post-menopausal and has a long history of diabetes. Which of the following would be the most important baseline test to undertake:

A  a full blood count
B  liver function tests
C  creatinine clearance
D  nerve conduction studies
E  a chest X-ray.

**186** You are asked to review a 15-year-old girl who is 28 days post stem-cell transplant for refractory acute lymphocytic leukaemia (ALL). She has developed acute graft-vs-host disease (GVHD) with hepatitis, gastrointestinal bleeding and skin signs. The haematology team have recently started her on systemic tacrolimus. What important potential side effect should be closely monitored for whilst she is taking the medication:

A   anaemia
B   polycythaemia
C   raised serum creatinine
D   hypertrichosis
E   methaemoglobinaemia.

**187** You are referred a patient who has recently emigrated from Germany. His psoriasis has been controlled for a number of years with fumaric acid esters (Fumaderm). The patient asks if the medication may be responsible for his flushing. What is the correct response:

A   it is definitely the cause of his flushing
B   flushing is a well recognised side effect of fumaric acid ester therapy
C   flushing is a rare but known side effect of fumaric acid ester therapy
D   flushing has not been reported as a side effect of fumaric acid therapy
E   it is definitely not the cause of his flushing.

**188** A 28-year-old woman presents as an emergency. She is known to you with biopsy proven gestational pemphigoid and is being treated with 80 mg/day of oral prednisolone. Over the last 24 hours she has developed intractable vomiting and feels extremely unwell. What dose of subcutaneous dexamethasone would you prescribe the patient as an equivalent to the dose of oral prednisolone:

A   12 mg
B   4 mg
C   80 mg
D   20 mg
E   160 mg.

**189** You review a patient with widespread tinea versicolor. Which of the following treatment options would not be appropriate:

A   topical ketoconazole
B   systemic itraconazole
C   topical selenium sulphide
D   topical miconazole
E   systemic griseofulvin.

**190** You review a 34-year-old man with recurrent tinea pedis. Despite regular treatment with topical miconazole and increased foot hygine he is still getting episodes of infection. There is no clinical or mycological evidence of onychomycosis. You decide to treat the patient with systemic terbinafine, what regime would you prescribe:

A   250 mg once daily for 4 weeks
B   500 mg one off dose
C   125 mg pulsed weekly every second week for 3 months
D   50 mg twice daily for 2 weeks
E   1 g twice daily for 6 weeks.

**191** You review a 41-year-old woman with moderate chronic plaque psoriasis. You plan to book her for psoralen plus ultraviolet A (PUVA) photochemotherapy. Which of her medications may affect her treatment:

A   codeine phosphate
B   oral contraceptive pill
C   omeprazole
D   doxycycline
E   atorvastatin.

**192** You see a 68-year-old woman in clinic who has longstanding chronic plaque psoriasis. She has been on methotrexate for many years but this was recently stopped due to a persistently raised pro-collagen III-NP. You want to start her on a biological agent, which of the following is a chimeric monoclonal antibody:

A   etanercept
B   infliximab
C   alefacept
D   ustekinumab
E   efalizumab.

**193** You want to start a 31-year-old woman on a biological agent for treatment resistant chronic plaque psoriasis. Her blood tests show a baseline lymphopenia. Which agent should you not prescribe this patient:

A   etanercept
B   adalimumab
C   alefacept
D   ustekinumab
E   efalizumab.

**194** An eight-year-old girl presents with an exacerbation of atopic eczema. You want to treat her with a moderate strength topical steroid ointment. Which of the following commercially available preparations would be appropriate:

A   fluocinolone acetonide 0.0025%
B   clobetasone butyrate 0.05%
C   mometasone furoate 0.1%
D   clobetasol propionate 0.05%
E   hydrocortisone butyrate 0.1%.

**195** Which of the following is a well recognised nail change that may occur with chemotherapy:

A   periungual pyogenic granulomas and paronychia
B   median nail dystrophy

C   onychogryphosis
D   Hallopeau's acrodermatitis
E   subungual exostosis.

**196** A 52-year-old man presents to his general practitioner with a widespread, symmetrical exanthem consistent with a drug reaction. Which of his medications is the most likely culprit:

A   aspirin
B   dapsone
C   amiodarone
D   ibuprofen
E   cefalexin.

**197** A 71-year-old man presents with a well defined oval patch on his leg. His general practitioner suspected a drug reaction and after stopping all his drugs the patch disappeared. When the patient was restarted on his medications the patch recurred in the same place. You suspect the patient has a fixed drug eruption, which of his medications is the likely culprit:

A   simvastatin
B   atenolol
C   doxycycline
D   omeprazole
E   captopril.

**198** A 79-year-old woman presents with numerous thick-walled blisters and urticated plaques suspicious of bullous pemphigoid. The patient asks if any of her medications may be responsible. Which of her medications is most likely to have precipitated her bullous pemphigoid:

A   methotrexate
B   chlorpromazine
C   mepacrine
D   furosemide
E   ramipril.

**199** A 48-year-old woman presents with an acneiform eruption and granulomatous plaques. She has recently been treated for thyrotoxicosis with radioiodine. You suspect that she has halogenoderma. Which of the following is a cause of halogenoderma:

A   ciclosporin
B   prednisolone
C   montelukast
D   phenytoin
E   amiodarone.

**200** A 67-year-old man presents acutely unwell with fever and rash. On examination he has widespread areas of symmetrical erythema with multiple small, non-follicular, sterile pustules. He was recently started on terbinafine for mycology proven onychomycosis. He has no personal or family history of psoriasis. What is the most likely diagnosis:

A   acute generalised pustular psoriasis
B   subcorneal pustulosis
C   acute generalised exanthematous pustulosis (AGEP)
D   bacterial folliculitis
E   candidal folliculitis.

**201** You are asked to see a six-year-old boy who is on the paediatric intensive care unit following cardiac surgery. He has developed a widespread papulopustular skin eruption with fever, hepatitis and eosinophilia. The cardiologists suspect the patient has developed drug reaction with eosinophilia and systemic symptoms (DRESS). Which of his medications is most likely to be responsible:

A   ramipril, taken for 3 months
B   trimethoprim, taken for 6 days
C   aciclovir, taken for 14 days
D   propranolol, taken for 6 months
E   aspirin, taken for 6 months.

**202** A patient presents with a widespread, biopsy proven lichenoid eruption. You suspect a lichenoid drug reaction, which of the following medications is most likely to have caused the reaction:

A   citalopram
B   cetirizine
C   gold
D   sodium valporate
E   dapsone.

# ANSWERS

## 176 D. Irreversible oligozoospermia

Methotrexate irreversibly inhibits the enzyme dihydrofolate reductase preventing the formation of the active metabolite tetrahydrofolate. It also has effects on purine metabolism and T-cell inhibition. Weekly, low dose methotrexate is used in a number of dermatological conditions including psoriasis. An initial test dose of 2.5–10 mg is given to check for pancytopenia, standard dosing is 10–20 mg once weekly.

Side effects include pancytopenia, hepatotoxicity, photosensitivity, alopecia, lung fibrosis and nausea. Oral ulceration is a sign of overdose and can be treated with folinic acid. Methotrexate causes a reversible oligozoospermia.

Absolute contraindications include pregnancy and breastfeeding. Relative contraindications are liver disease, alcohol excess, active infection and immunodeficiency.

Interactions are seen with a number of medications. Sulphonamides inhibit the folate pathway acting synergistically with methotrexate to cause pancytopenia. Alcohol and retinoids cause concomitant liver damage and should be avoided. Probenecid and dipyridamole may lead to intracellular accumulation of methotrexate. Other potential interacting agents include non-steroidal anti- inflammatory medications, furosemide, chloramphenicol, tetracyclines, phenytoin and phenothiazines.

In this question the patient may be counselled about reversible, but not irreversible oligozoospermia.

## 177 D. Continue with the same dose of methotrexate and repeat the test in 3 months

Pro-collagen III NP assays are an accepted marker of liver fibrosis in psoriatic patients taking methotrexate. The assay is not helpful in patients with significant inflammatory arthropathy. Guidelines suggest that serum pro-collagen III NP levels should be measured before starting methotrexate and every 2–3 months during treatment. The normal range for pro-collagen III NP is 1.7–4.2.

Indications for considering a liver biopsy:
- pre-treatment level above 8.0
- level above 4.2 in three samples within 12 months
- level above 8.0 in two consecutive samples.

Indications for consideration of withdrawal of methotrexate:
• level above 10 in three samples within 12 months.
In this question the patient has an isolated mildly raised pro-collagen III NP level, an appropriate course of action would be to continue with the methotrexate and repeat the test in 2–3 months.

## 178 E. Increase the dose of hydroxycarbamide to 500 mg twice daily

Hydroxycarbamide is also known as hydroxyurea, it is primarily used in haematological malignancies but it also helpful in a number of dermatological conditions including psoriasis. The precise mechanism of action is not known, it has effects on deoxyribonucleotide production, nitric oxide levels and foetal haemoglobin production. Patients are normally started on a dose of 500 mg once daily and increased to a maximum of 2 g per day.

Side effects are mostly due to effects on red blood cells. All patients develop a megaloblastosis and drop their haemoglobin level by 1 to 2 g/dL. Less commonly patients may develop frank anaemia, thrombocytopenia and leucopenia. The medication should be stopped if the haemoglobin level drops by more than 3 g/dL, the white cell count drops below 4.0 x10⁹/L or the platelet count drops below 100 x10⁹/L. Other side effects include a reversible hepatitis, leg ulceration and hyperpigmentation.

Absolute contraindications include pregnancy and breastfeeding. Relative contraindications include cardiac, pulmonary or renal disease and blood dyscrasias.

The only significant drug interaction is synergy with the chemotherapeutic agent cytarabine.

In this question the patient has developed a megaloblastic anaemia with a drop in HB by 1.6 g/dL. This is within the expected physiological response to hydroxycarbamide. As the patient has started to show a clinical response to the drug it is reasonable to increase the dose.

## 179 B. 250 mg per day

Azathioprine is an immunosuppressant drug used in organ transplantation and a number of autoimmune disorders. In dermatology it is most commonly used for severe eczema and immunobullous disorders. It works by inhibiting purine synthesis thereby reducing the proliferation of leukocytes. Patients are normally started on 50 mg/day increasing to a maximum of 2.5 mg/kg/day.

The primary side effect of concern is pancytopenia, this may be predicted by measuring the TPMT enzyme activity and a dose reduction may be used:

**Table 10.1** Dosing of azathioprine according to TMPT activity

| TPMT level | Maximum safe dose of azathioprine |
| --- | --- |
| Less than 5 U | Drug is contraindicated |
| 5–14 U | 0.5 mg/kg/day |
| 15–19 U | 1.5 mg/kg/day |
| Greater than 19 U | 2.5 mg/kg/day |

Other side effects include a long term risk of haematological and cutaneous malignancy and a rare hypersensitivity reaction.

A dose reduction of azathioprine is needed in patients with renal impairment:

**Table 10.2** Dosing of azathioprine according to renal function

| Glomerular filtration rate (GFR) | Dose reduction of azathioprine |
| --- | --- |
| ↓10 mls/min | 50% dose reduction |
| 10–50 mls/min | 25% dose reduction |
| Over 50 mls/min | No dose reduction |

The only absolute contraindication is a previous hypersensitivity reaction. Relative contraindications include pregnancy and active infection. Drug interactions are seen with allopurinol and captopril both of which may increase the risk of pancytopenia. Azathioprine reduces the effectiveness of muscle relaxants and warfarin.

In this case the patient has normal TPMT activity and no other contraindications, a suitable maximum dose would be 2.5 mg/kg/day.

**180 A. Continue isotretinoin and add in prednisolone 40 mg/day**
Retinoids are a group of drugs closely related to vitamin A. They have a number of effects on the body including regulation of epithelial cell growth. In dermatology commonly used retinoids include those shown in Table 10.3.

**Table 10.3** Retinoids used in dermatology

| Retinoid | Generation | Use |
| --- | --- | --- |
| Tretinoin | First generation | Topically in acne and anti-ageing products |
| Isotretinoin | First generation | Systemically for acne and hidradenitis suppurativa |
| Alitretinoin | First generation | Systemically for hand eczema |
| Etretinate | Second generation | Systemically for psoriasis, now rarely used |
| Acitretin | Second generation | Systemically for psoriasis, a metabolite of etretinate |
| Tarazotene | Third generation | Topically for psoriasis and acne |
| Bexarotene | Third generation | Systemically for cutaneous lymphoma |
| Adapalene | Third generation | Topically for acne |

The most important side effect of retinoids is their potent teratogenicity, in many countries comprehensive pregnancy prevention programs are used for women of childbearing age. Other side effects include a dose dependant cheilitis, epistaxis, dry mouth, xerosis, pruritus, skin fragility, photosensitivity, alopecia, pyogenic granuloma formation and nail changes. Bone pain may occur with or without bony exotosis, myalgia and arthralgia. Transiently raised liver function tests and serum lipids are also seen.

The potential psychiatric side effects of systemic retinoids are controversial and care should be taken when prescribing for patients with a history of depression or suicidal ideation.

Due to its potent teratogenicity pregnancy, contemplation of pregnancy and breastfeeding are absolute contraindications. Relative contraindications include leucopenia, hypercholesterolaemia, hypertriglyceridaemia, significant hepatic or renal dysfunction and hypothyroidism.

Interactions are seen with tetracyclines which act synergistically to cause raised intracranial pressure. Concurrent alcohol or methotrexate use increases the risk of hepatotoxicity. Macrolide antibiotics and azole antifungals increase serum retinoid levels whereas anticonvulsants decrease serum levels. Vitamin A supplements should be avoided when taking a systemic retinoid.

In this case the patient has developed pyogenic granulomas and systemic upset after starting isotretinoin. Appropriate treatment would be to continue the isotretinoin at the same dose and add in a systemic corticosteroid. As the patient improves the steroids can be tapered and the isotretinoin increased to 1 mg/kg/day.

## 181 C. Propranolol

Ciclosporin A is a fungally derived immunosuppressant that binds to cyclophilin on the cell surface of immunocompetent T-lymphocytes. This in turn inhibits calcineurin a transcription factor for interleukin 2. Ciclosporin is used as an anti-rejection drug after organ transplantation and for inflammatory skin conditions such as eczema and psoriasis. It is usually started at a dose of 2.5 mg/kg/day and increased to a maximum of 5 mg/kg/day.

The most common side effects are hypertension and renal impairment. All patients should have two baseline blood pressure and creatinine readings and regular monitoring whilst taking the medication. Nephrotoxicity is initially reversible but becomes irreversible after 1–2 years. If serum creatinine is raised greater than 25% from baseline a dose reduction of 25–50% should be used, if serum creatinine rises to over 50% from baseline the medication should be discontinued. Ciclosporin related hypertension is often mild, transient and can be managed with anti-hypertensives. Long term use of ciclosporin carries an increased risk of cancer in particular SCC and lymphoma. Other side effects include gum hypertrophy, hepatotoxicity, myositis, hyperlipidaemia and hypertrichosis.

Absolute contraindications include severe baseline renal impairment and uncontrolled hypertension. Relative contraindications are hypertension, use in children and use in the elderly.

Ciclosporin has a number of drug interactions. Plasma levels may be increased by simvastatin, danazol, diltiazem, verapamil, nicardipine, azole antifungals, quinolone antibiotics, erythromycin, trimethoprim, co-trimoxazole, grapefruit juice, amphotericin and aminoglycosides. Plasma levels may be reduced by rifampicin, isoniazid, phenytoin, phenobarbitone and carbamazepine. There is an increased risk of hyperkalaemia when using ACE inhibitors, potassium sparing diuretics and potassium supplements. Nifedipine has a synergistic effect causing gum hypertrophy and should be avoided.

In this question the drug of choice would be propranolol which has no significant interactions with ciclosporin. Ramipril and spironolactone both carry an increased risk of hyperkalaemia when used with ciclosporin. Diltiazem and verapamil increase plasma ciclosporin levels.

## 182 E. Intravenous methylene blue and oxygen

Dapsone was developed as an antibacterial sharing many similarities with the sulphonamide group of antibiotics. It works by inhibiting bacterial synthesis of dihydrofolic acid. The mechanism of action in skin disorders is less well understood. It is primarily used in immunobullous disorders but has a wide spectrum of action in many inflammatory dermatosis including acne and cutaneous lupus. It is normally started at a dose of 50 mg/day and increased to a maximum of 300 mg/day.

Common side effects include dose dependant methaemoglobinaemia and haemolysis that may be exacerbated in patients with Glucose-6-phosphate dehydrogenase (G6PD) deficiency. Less commonly patients may develop agranulocytosis, photosensitivity, hepatitis and peripheral neuropathy. A rare dapsone hypersensitivity syndrome may occur with fever, hepatitis and a generalised exanthem.

The only absolute contraindication is prior hypersensitivity. Relative contraindications include low G6PD levels, significant cardiac or lung disease and allergy to sulphonamides. It is probably safe in pregnancy and lactation.

Interactions are seen with probenecid, trimethoprim and methotrexate which increase serum dapsone levels. Charcoal, rifampicin and para-aminobenzoic acid (PABA) reduce serum dapsone levels. Sulphonamides and anti-malarial drugs may exacerbate any haemolysis.

In this question the patient has developed a significant methaemoglobinaemia of 40% which requires urgent treatment. Methaemoglobin levels below 15% are often asymptomatic and levels above 70% may be fatal. The methaemoglobinaemia is likely to be related to the patient's dapsone therapy and a possible underlying diagnosis of G6PD deficiency. Treatment of methaemoglobinaemia is with methylene blue and oxygen, amyl nitrate is likely to exacerbate the problem.

## 183 A. Ocular toxicity

Anti-malarial drugs are most commonly used by dermatologists to treat cutaneous lupus and porphyria. Hydroxychloroquine decreases lysosomal pH in antigen presenting cells and blockades toll-like receptors, it is given at a dose of 200–400 mg/day. Chloroquine inhibits lymphocyte proliferation and the production of IL-1, it is given at a dose of 250–300 mg/day. Mepacrine is a synthetic substitute for quinine, it is given at a dose of 100–200 mg/day.

The most serious side effect of anti-malarial drug therapy is an irreversible retinopathy which is most commonly seen with chloroquine. Haemolysis may occur in patients with G6PD deficiency. Rashes of various morphologies are common as is blue-black hyperpigmentation. Some patients develop a reversible bleaching of their hair. Long term use of mepacrine can lead to yellow discolouration of the skin. All anti-malarial drugs have the potential to exacerbate psoriasis.

Relative contraindications include blood dyscrasias, hepatic disorders and retinal pathology. Hydroxychloroquine is considered to be the safest anti-malarial medication in pregnancy and lactation.

Interactions occur with cimetidine which raises serum anti-malarial drug levels. Kaolin and magnesium trisilicate may reduce the absorption of anti-malarials drugs and anti-malarials drugs may increase serum digoxin levels.

In this question anti-malarial drugs should not be combined due to the risk of synergistic ocular toxicity. Anti-malarial drugs are not especially hepatotoxic and they cause hyperpigmentation not hypopigmentation. Haemolysis may occur but is rare and although anti-malarial drugs may worsen psoriasis they are unlikely to precipitate pustular psoriasis in a patient with no history of the disease.

### 184 B. Gastrointestinal upset

Mycophenolate mofetil is a prodrug for the active metabolite mycophenolic acid. It is fungally derived and works by blocking purine synthesis in B and T lymphocytes. Primarily used as an immunosuppressant in organ transplant recipients it is also effective in a number of cutaneous disorders including pemphigus vulgaris, lupus and psoriasis. It is normally given in a dose of 2 g/day increasing to a maximum of 3 g/day.

Gastrointestinal side effects are common. Infections, leucopenia and anaemia are also seen. Less commonly thrombophlebitis, thrombosis, gastritis, pure red cell aplasia and progressive multifocal leukoencephalopathy may occur.

Pregnancy and allergy to mycophenolate are absolute contraindications. Relative contraindications include breastfeeding, peptic ulceration, hepatic, renal and cardiovascular disease.

Drug interactions are seen with cholestyramine, iron hydroxide, aluminium hydroxide and magnesium hydroxide which all reduce serum mycophenolate levels. Serum aciclovir levels may also be raised when given concurrently with mycophenolate.

In this question the most common side effect seen with mycophenolate mofetil therapy is gastrointestinal upset. Anaemia, thrombophlebitis and progressive multifocal leukoencephalopathy are less commonly seen side effects, renal failure is not seen.

### 185 D. Nerve conduction studies
Thalidomide is a derivative of glutamic acid, it has anti-inflammatory, immunomodulatory and anti-angiogenic properties. Developed as a sedative it is now used in myeloma, erythema nodosum leprosy and a number of off-licence dermatological conditions. Dosing is started at 50–100 mg/day and increased to a maximum of 300 mg/day.

The most serious side effect of thalidomide is potent teratogenicity. Very serious consideration must be undertaken before prescribing the medication to women of childbearing age. A dose related peripheral sensory neuropathy may also occur and it is recommended that baseline and monitoring neurological examination and nerve conduction studies are undertaken on all patients taking the medication. Other side effects include sedation, constipation, ovarian failure, leucopenia and erythroderma.

Absolute contraindications include pregnancy, consideration of pregnancy, inadequate contraception in a sexually active fertile female, breastfeeding and peripheral neuropathy. Relative contraindications include cardiac, renal and liver disease or a history of thrombosis.

No serious drug interactions are seen. The sedative effect of thalidomide may be synergistic when used with other sedatives such as alcohol, barbiturates or phenothiazines.

In this question the most important baseline test would be nerve conduction studies. The patient has a history of diabetes and may have a diabetes related peripheral neuropathy, if so this would be a contraindication for treatment with thalidomide. A full blood count, liver function tests and serum urea and creatinine levels are recommended baseline blood tests. Creatinine clearance and a chest X-ray are not required.

### 186 C. Raised serum creatinine
Tacrolimus is a macrolide with a similar structure and mechanism of action to ciclosporin. It blocks the action of calcineurin and other

cytokines such as IL-8. It is primarily used to prevent organ rejection after transplantation and for treatment of GVHD. It was hoped that the drug would be effective in a number of dermatological disorders but its use has been limited due to side effects. Topically tacrolimus is licensed for use in atopic eczema. When given systemically a dose of 1 to 2 mg/day is often used with dose adjustment depending on serum levels.

The side effect profile is similar to ciclosporin with renal impairment and hypertension often limiting the use of the drug. Diabetes is more commonly seen with tacrolimus and hypertrichosis occurs less frequently than with ciclosporin.

Hypersensitivity to the drug and pregnancy are absolute contraindications. It should be avoided when breastfeeding.

Interactions are seen with a number of medications. Synergistic nephrotoxicity is seen with ciclosporin, NSAIDs and rifampicin. Hyperkalaemia may occur with angiotensin II receptor blockers, potassium sparing diuretics and potassium supplements. Increased plasma concentrations of tacrolimus may be seen with macrolide antibiotics, azole antifungals, calcium channel blockers and omeprazole. Reduced plasma concentrations may occur with phenytoin and phenobarbital.

In the question, the most important potential side effect to monitor for would be a raised serum creatinine; the patient would also be closely monitored for hypertension. Hypertrichosis is less common than with ciclosporin and haematological side effects are rare.

### 187 B. Flushing is a well recognised side effect of fumaric acid ester therapy

Fumaric acid esters are a popular choice for treatment resistant psoriasis in central Europe. The active compound fumaric acid is an intermediate in the citric acid and urea cycles. It has effects on keratinocyte proliferation and activation. Dosing is dependent on the commercially available mixture of fumaric acid esters.

The most common side effect is gastrointestinal upset which occurs in up to two-thirds of patients. Flushing is also common occurring in one third of patients. Other side effects include lymphopenia and eosinophilia. There are conflicting reports on whether renal impairment is seen.

Little is known about fumaric acid esters drug interactions although it is recommended that patients should not receive concurrent immunosuppressants or nephrotoxic agents.

## 188 A. 12 mg

Systemic corticosteroids are widely used for a variety of dermatological conditions due to their potent anti-inflammatory and immunosuppressive actions. The use of steroids tends only to be limited by their side effects. The dose of steroid used depends on the drug's potency, patient's weight and desired effects.

**Table 10.4** Equivalent doses of commonly used systemic corticosteroids

| Steroid | Dose |
| --- | --- |
| Prednisolone | 10 mg |
| Hydrocortisone | 40 mg |
| Triamcinolone | 8 mg |
| Dexamethasone | 1.5 mg |

Side effects of systemic corticosteroid therapy:
- cardiovascular – hypertension, fluid retention and oedema
- musculoskeletal – osteoporosis, osteonecrosis, poor growth (children), redistribution of fat
- gastrointestinal – peptic ulcer disease, gastritis, oesophagitis
- psychiatric – psychosis, mood change
- other – obesity, hyperlipidaemia, hyperglycaemia, amenorrhoea, infections, acne, hirsutism, leukocytosis, striae.

Patients taking long term corticosteroids should carry a steroid card as rapid withdrawal of exogenous steroids can lead to a potentially fatal adrenal crisis.

There are a number of contraindications for the use of systemic steroid therapy – active tuberculosis, systemic fungal infections, active peptic ulcer disease, severe psychiatric illness and uncontrolled diabetes. In dermatology an important contraindication is an extensive chronic dermatosis (e.g. psoriasis) which is likely to rebound when therapy is stopped.

Drug interactions are seen with medications that affect the cytochrome P450 microsomal enzyme system.

**Table 10.5** Drug interactions with the cytochrome P450 pathway and their effect on corticosteroid clearance

|  | Cytochrome P450 inducers | Cytochrome P450 inhibitors |
|---|---|---|
| Interacting medications | Phenytoin, carbamazepine, barbiturates, rifampicin, alcohol, sulphonylureas (PC-BRAS) | Omeprazole, disulfiram, erythromycin, valporate, isoniazid, cimetidine, ethanol, sulphonamides (ODEVICES) |
| Effects on corticosteroid clearance | Increases the clearance of corticosteroids | Reduces the clearance of corticosteroids |
| Clinical significance | An increased dose of corticosteroid may be required | A decreased dose of corticosteroid may be required |

In this question the patient was taking 80 mg/day of prednisolone, as 10 mg of prednisolone has a similar potency to 1.5 mg of dexamethasone, 80 mg of prednisolone is the equivalent of 12 mg of dexamethasone.

### 189 E. Systemic griseofulvin

Griseofulvin is a fungiostatic antifungal that disrupts the mitotic spindle of dermatophytes inhibiting mitosis. Adult dosing is 500 mg once or twice daily, in children 10–20 mg/kg/day.

Side effects include gastrointestinal upset, headache, hepatotoxicity, peripheral neuropathy, leucopoenia and drug induced lupus.

Contraindications include severe liver disease, lupus, porphyria, pregnancy and breastfeeding.

Interactions are seen with primidone and barbiturates which reduce the absorption of griseofulvin. Griseofulvin may reduce the effect of warfarin, reduce serum ciclosporin levels and increase the metabolism of oestrogen and progesterone affecting the oral contraceptive pill.

In this question the patient has a superficial skin infection with malassezia furfur. Topical and systemic azole antifungals and selenium sulphide have good activity against this yeast. Systemic griseofulvin has no activity against malassezia or candida infections.

**Table 10.6** Activity spectra of commonly used systemic antifungal agents

| Antifungal | Activity |
|---|---|
| Terbinafine | Good activity against common dermatophytes – onychomycosis, superficial tinea infections |

*continued*

| Griseofulvin | Good activity against common dermatophytes – tinea capitis, onychomycosis, not effective against malassezia or candida |
| --- | --- |
| Itraconazole | Effective against dermatophytes, yeasts and some moulds |
| Fluconazole | Primarily used for systemic candida infection, also effective against common dermatophytes |
| Ketoconazole | Effective against most dermatophytes and candida, limited use due to potential fatal hepatotoxicity |
| Voriconazole | Used for invasive aspergillosis, candidiasis and fusarium |
| Amphotericin B | Used for disseminated systemic fungal and yeast infections, risk of anaphylaxis on first dose |

## 190 A. 250 mg once daily for 4 weeks

Terbinafine is a fungiostatic antifungal that inhibits squalene epoxidase, a vital component of fungal cell membrane synthesis. Adult dose of terbinafine is 250 mg once daily, doses for children vary from 62.5 mg–250 mg depending on the child's weight.

Side effects of terbinafine include gastrointestinal upset, headache, rash, hepatotoxicity and drug induced lupus. It may also cause an exacerbation of psoriasis.

Contraindications include widespread psoriasis, autoimmune disease, renal or hepatic disease pregnancy and breastfeeding.

Drug interactions are seen with rifampicin which reduces plasma terbinafine levels and cimetidine which increases plasma terbinafine levels. Effects on oestrogen and progesterone may interfere with the oral contraceptive pill.

In this question the patient requires an adult dose of terbinafine which is 250 mg once daily. Superficial dermatophyte infections such as tinea pedis are treated for 2–6 weeks. Onychomycosis is treated for 3–6 months.

## 191 D. Doxycycline

Psoralens are plant derived chemicals that lead to a cutaneous phototoxic reaction when exposed to UV radiation. The psoralen 8-methoxypsoralen (8-MOP) is often used with UVA radiation to treat psoriasis (PUVA) along with a large number of other dermatological conditions. Psoralens may be directly applied to the skin or taken systemically. When exposed to UV radiation psoralens have a number of local effects including suppression of DNA synthesis, immunosuppression, selective cytotoxicity and stimulation of melanocytes.

Side effects of PUVA can be split into short term and long term effects:

- short term – phototoxic reactions, gastrointestinal upset, CNS disturbance, bronchoconstriction, hepatotoxicity, exanthems
- long term – photoaging of the skin, non-melanoma and melanoma skin cancer, cataracts.

Absolute contraindications include pemphigus, pemphigoid, lupus with photosensitivity, xeroderma pigmentosum and lactation. Relative contraindications include photosensitising medications, history of skin cancer, photodamaged skin, pregnancy and severe cardiac, liver or renal disease.

Drug interactions are rarely seen. There is a theoretical risk that cytochrome P450 inducers (*see* question 188) enhance the metabolism of psoralens thereby reducing their effectiveness. Photosensitising drugs may have a synergistic effect leading to phototoxic reactions.

In this question doxycycline stands out as a potential photosensitizing medication. Although taking photosensitising medications is not a contraindication to PUVA a dose reduction in UVA may be required.

Phototoxic medications lead to an exaggerated sunburn-like response after exposure to UV radiation. Examples include:

- fluoroquinolones, tetracyclines
- amiodarone
- furosemide, thiazides
- atenolol, captopril, nifedipine
- NSAIDs
- phenothiazines
- psoralens (topically, systemically, medication or plant derived).

Photoallergic medications lead to an eczematous, pruritic rash after exposure to UV radiation. Examples include:

- topical sunscreens and fragrances
- topical antibiotics and NSAIDs
- quinidine
- quinolones
- griseofulvin
- NSAIDs
- sulphonamides.

## 192 B. Infliximab

The introduction of biological agents has transformed the treatment of severe psoriasis. The use of these agents has only been limited by their high cost. In the UK strict criteria must be met before a patient is eligible for treatment with a biological agent.

- Severe psoriasis for over 6 months with a Psoriasis Area and Severity Index (PASI) greater than 10 and a Dermatology Life Quality Index (DLQI) greater than 10, and one of:
  - have developed, or are at risk of developing drug related toxicity from a systemic therapy for psoriasis
  - intolerance of or contraindicated for standard systemic therapies
  - poor clinical response to standard systemic therapies
  - repeated inpatient admissions due to psoriasis
  - severe, unstable or life threatening psoriasis.

A patient may also meet the criteria for a biological agent due to associated psoriatic arthropathy.

**Table 10.7** Biological agents used in psoriasis

| Name (trade name) | Structure and mechanism of action | Standard dose |
| --- | --- | --- |
| Etanercept (Enbrel) | Fully human, anti-TNF monoclonal antibody | 25 mg or 50 mg twice weekly or 50 mg once weekly |
| Infliximab (Remicade) | Chimeric (25% mouse, 75% human), anti-TNF monoclonal antibody | 5 mg/kg, at baseline, 2 weeks, 6 weeks then 8–12 weekly |
| Adalimumab (Humira) | Fully human, anti-TNF monoclonal antibody | 1st dose 80 mg then 40 mg every 2 weeks |
| Alefacept (Amevive) | Fully human, inhibitor of CD2 and LFA-3 | 15 mg weekly |
| Efalizumab* (Raptiva) | Fully human, inhibitor of CD11a | 1 mg/kg weekly |
| Ustekinumab (Stelara) | Fully human, inhibitor of IL-12 and IL-23 | 45 mg at baseline, week 4 and week 12 then 12 weekly |

*Efalizumab was withdrawn in February 2009 after 3 patients developed progressive multifocal leukoencephalopathy.

In this question infliximab is the only chimeric monoclonal antibody, this may account for the higher rates of antibody formation against the drug.

**193 C. Alefacept**

Biological therapies have a number of side effects:

- injection site reactions occur with all biologic agents but are most commonly seen with etanercept, they are rarely serious
- all biological agents carry a small increased risk of malignancy, especially lymphoma
- there is an increased risk of infection and serious infection with all biological agents, reactivation of latent tuberculosis is well recognised
- anti-TNF biological agents are associated with new onset demyelinating disorders and exacerbation of pre-existing multiple sclerosis
- some patients develop ANA antibodies whilst on biological therapies, only rarely does this lead to a drug induced lupus which tends to resolve on stopping the medication
- patients may develop antibodies to the biological agents but this is only clinically relevant for infliximab where antibodies are associated with an increased risk of infusion reactions and reduced efficacy
- 20% of patients on infliximab develop non-serious infusion reactions such as headache, flushing and nausea; 1% develop serious reactions such as anaphylaxis, hypotension and chest pain
- adalimumab can be associated with leucopenia and thrombocytopenia, alefacept with lymphopenia and efalizumab with thrombocytopenia.

Absolute contraindications include sensitivity to the drug, pregnancy and active or chronic infection. Relative contraindications include a family or personal history of demyelinating diseases, history of malignancy and concomitant immunosuppressive treatment. Congestive cardiac failure is a contraindication for infliximab and etanercept. Thrombocytopenia is a contraindication for treatment with efalizumab and lymphopenia is a contraindication for using alefacept.

Drug interactions are rarely seen with biological agents. Patients should avoid co-administration with the IL-1 antagonist anakinra due to a synergistic increased risk of infection. Methotrexate reduces the clearance of adalimumab but this does not seem to be clinically relevant. Patients treated with biologic agents should not receive live vaccines.

In this question the patient has a baseline lymphopenia and should avoid alefacept.

## 194 B. Clobetasone butyrate 0.05%
Commonly used commercially available topical steroid preparations are shown in Table 10.8.

**Table 10.8** Commercially available topical steroid preparations

| Steroid | Brand name | Strength |
| --- | --- | --- |
| Hydrocortisone 0.5% to 1% | – | Mild |
| Fluocinolone acetonide 0.0025% | Synalar 1:10 | Mild |
| Clobetasone butyrate 0.05% | Eumovate, Trimovate | Moderate |
| Betamethasone valerate 0.025% | Betnovate-RD | Moderate |
| Alclometasone dipropionate 0.05% | Modrasone | Moderate |
| Fludroxycortide 0.0125% | Halean | Moderate |
| Fluocinolone acetonide 0.00625% | Synalar 1:4 | Moderate |
| Betamethasone valerate 0.1% | Betnovate | Potent |
| Hydrocortisone butyrate 0.1% | Locoid | Potent |
| Diflucortolone valerate 0.1% | Nerisone | Potent |
| Fluocinolone acetonide 0.025% | Synalar | Potent |
| Fluocinonide 0.05% | Metosyn | Potent |
| Mometasone furoate 0.1% | Elocon | Potent |
| Triamcinolone acetonide 0.1% | Tri-adacortyl | Potent |
| Clobetasol propionate 0.05% | Dermovate | Super potent |
| Diflucortolone valerate 0.3% | Nerisone forte | Super potent |

In this question clobetasone butyrate would be an appropriate moderate strength steroid ointment to use in this patient.

## 195 A. Periungual pyogenic granulomas and paronychia
A number of nail changes may be seen when patients are treated with chemotherapy:
- Beau's lines
- onychomadesis
- periungual pyogenic granulomas
- true and apparent leukonychia
- nail thinning and brittleness
- onycholysis and photo-onycholysis

- melanonychia.

Periungual pyogenic granulomas may also be seen with:

- retinoids
- gefitinib
- cetuximab
- indinavir
- lamivudine
- methotrexate.

Median nail dystrophy is often due to a habitual tic, onychogryphosis and subungual exostosis are due to repetitive trauma and Hallopeau's acrodermatitis is associated with psoriasis.

## 196 E. Cefalexin

Most drug reactions are due to the development of hypersensitisation to the drug or a component of the drug. Sometimes they can show cross sensitisation, for example with penicillins and cephalosporins.

Common causes of a drug exanthem:

- penicillins, cephalosporins, sulphonamides
- anticonvulsants
- allopurinol.

Patients may also develop drug sensitivity that may present as a type 1 reaction with anaphylaxis or urticaria.

Common causes of an anaphylactic/urticarial drug reaction:

- penicillins, cephalosporins, sulphonamides, tetracyclines
- NSAIDs
- contrast media
- monoclonal antibodies
- ACE inhibitors.

It is important to distinguish this reaction from drugs that exacerbate idiopathic urticaria such as:

- aspirin
- opiates
- NSAIDs
- alcohol.

Some patients may develop an erythrodermic drug reaction, common causes are:

- allopurinol
- beta-lactam antibiotics, sulphonamides
- anticonvulsants

- gold
- sulphasalazine
- furosemide.

## 197 C. Doxycycline

This patient has a history typical of a fixed drug eruption. Patients present with a fixed oval patch or plaque that recurs in the same place every time the drug is taken. With repeated attacks more lesions can appear, postinflammatory hyperpigmentation is common.

Common causes of a fixed drug eruption:
- barbiturates, chlordiazepoxide,
- tetracyclines, metronidazole, sulphonamides
- NSAIDs, aspirin, paracetamol, oxyphenbutazone
- phenolphthalein (laxative)
- anti-malarial drugs.

In this case the most likely responsible drug is the tetracycline doxycycline.

## 198 D. Furosemide

Blistering is a well known manifestation of cutaneous drug reactions. The blistering may be secondary to a severe eczematous or urticarial drug reaction or it may be a primary drug reaction presenting as an immunobullous disorder, bullous erythema multiforme or porphyria cutanea tarda.

Common causes of drug induced bullous pemphigoid:
- furosemide
- paracetamol
- amoxicillin, ciprofloxacin, tetracyclines
- D-penicillamine
- potassium iodide
- gold
- captopril.

Common causes of drug induced pemphigus:
- penicillamine
- captopril
- rifampicin.

Common causes of drug induced linear IgA disease:
- vancomycin
- lithium
- captopril.

Common causes of drug induced pseudoporphyria:
- NSAIDs, especially naproxen
- furosemide
- tetracyclines.

In this question furosemide is a well recognised cause of a number of bullous drug reactions including bullous pemphigoid.

### 199 E. Amiodarone

Halogenodermas are rare dermatoses that present with acneiform eruptions, pustules, granulomatous plaques and ulcers. They occur following exposure to bromides, fluorides, iodides and iodine containing compounds. Treatment is withdrawal of the offending agent, corticosteroids and ciclosporin.

Drugs that may cause halogenoderma:
- radioiodine, potassium iodide, iodine supplements
- iodine containing contrast media and antiseptic agents
- amiodarone
- potassium bromide
- ipratropium bromide
- cough/cold remedies.

In this question the iodine containing medication amiodarone is the most likely to cause a halogenoderma.

### 200 C. Acute generalised exanthematous pustulosis (AGEP)

This patient is presenting with a typical history of acute generalised exanthematous pustulosis (AGEP), a rare drug reaction. Patients present with fever and numerous small, non-follicular, sterile pustules arising from large areas of oedematous, erythematous skin. The reaction often occurs within five days of starting a new medication, drugs are responsible for over 90% of cases of AGEP.

Common causes of AGEP:
- beta-lactam antibiotics, macrolides, metronidazole
- terbinafine
- calcium channel blockers
- hydroxychloroquine
- carbamazepine
- paracetamol.

In this question the widespread nature of the rash and systemic upset makes a folliculitis unlikely. There is no family or personal history of psoriasis which makes acute generalised pustular psoriasis less likely, although it is clinically difficult to distinguish this from AGEP. Subcorneal pustular dermatosis is a chronic relapsing condition that favours the flexural trunk and proximal extremities.

## 201 B. Trimethoprim, taken for 6 days
Drug Reaction with Eosinophilia and Systemic Symptoms (DRESS) is also known as drug hypersensitivity syndrome, patients present with:
- fever
- widespread papulopustular or erythematous rash
- systemic involvement – hepatitis, myocarditis, nephritis or pneumonitis
- eosinophilia and atypical lymphocytosis (~30% of cases).

Mortality from DRESS is between 5–10%. Treatment involves withdrawal of the offending drug and corticosteroids may be helpful in some cases.

Common causes of DRESS:
- allopurinol
- anticonvulsants
- sulphonamides, trimethoprim, minocycline
- anti-HIV medications
- gold
- dapsone.

In this question trimethoprim is the most likely precipitant of this patient's DRESS. Most reactions occur within 1–8 weeks of starting a new medication which makes ramipril, propranolol and aspirin unlikely. Aciclovir is not a well described cause of DRESS.

## 202 C. Gold
Lichenoid drug reactions may occur secondary to systemic medications where patients develop a skin rash typical of lichen planus.

Common causes of a lichenoid drug reaction:
- gold
- beta-blockers, ACE inhibitors, methyldopa
- anti-malarial drugs
- thiazides, furosemide, spironolactone
- penicillamine.

Patients may also develop an oral lichenoid reaction clinically indistinguishable from oral lichen planus. This is often due to a type IV contact allergy to dental amalgams and fillings.

Rarely, keratoderma may also present as a drug reaction, causes include:

- arsenic
- hydroxyurea
- lithium
- verapamil
- imatinib
- venlafaxine.

# Chapter 11

# Dermatopathology

## QUESTIONS

**203** Prior to seeing a patient on the haematology ward you review a histopathology report of an incisional skin biopsy taken earlier in the week. The report states that there are few diagnostic features on the biopsy: 'The epidermis is normal. In the upper dermis a sparse lymphocytic infiltrate is seen in a perivascular pattern. The reticular dermis and subcutaneous tissues are unremarkable.'

What is the most likely diagnosis:

A infiltrate of acute myelomonocytic leukaemia
B tumour stage mycosis fungoides
C erythema nodosum
D drug exanthema
E Sweet's syndrome.

**204** At the dermatopathology meeting you are discussing a difficult case with the pathologist. When reviewing the slide he points out an impressive band-like infiltrate of inflammatory cells at the dermal-epidermal junction. Of your original differential which is now the least likely diagnosis:

A granuloma annulare
B lupus
C lichenoid keratosis
D Bowen's disease
E lichen planus.

**205** You are called to review a one-year-old child admitted by the paediatric team for an exacerbation of asthma. The patient has a widespread rash which you biopsy. Three days later you contact the histopathologist as the patient is deteriorating. The haematoxylin and eosin (H&E) stain shows a diffuse dense infiltrate of monomorphous cells with basophilic granules throughout the dermis. Further stains have been ordered and are awaited. The most likely diagnosis is:

A   nummular eczema
B   lupus
C   lichen planus
D   erythema multiforme
E   mastocytosis.

**206** In clinic you see an emergency patient with a worsening rash. The patient gives a history of short lived blisters but on examination you see only superficial erosions. A biopsy is taken which shows a vesiculobullous pattern with a subcorneal split. What is the most likely diagnosis:

A   porphyria cutanea tarda
B   bullous pemphigoid
C   staphylococcal scalded skin syndrome
D   pemphigus vulgaris
E   bullous lupus.

**207** A middle-aged patient is admitted under the ENT team with a quinsy. Following surgical drainage and treatment with cephalosporin antibiotics the patient develops a widespread bullous rash. The initial skin biopsy shows a vesiculobullous pattern with a subepidermal split and lymphocytic infiltrate. What is the likely diagnosis:

A   bullous pemphigoid
B   bullous erythema multiforme
C   pemphigus foliaceus
D   pemphigus vulgaris
E   staphylococcal scalded skin syndrome.

**208** When reviewing a skin biopsy you see a dermal inflammatory infiltrate composed primarily of histiocytes. Which of the following differentials would be least likely:

A  xanthogranuloma
B  sarcoidosis
C  atypical mycobacterial infection
D  a ruptured hair follicle
E  dermatomyositis.

**209** At the dermatopathology meeting you are discussing a case with the pathologist. She comments on a collection of neutrophils in the epidermis and asks what this would look like clinically. What is the most likely appearance:

A  comedonal eruption
B  maculopapular exanthem
C  it is impossible to say
D  pustular rash
E  folliculitis.

**210** A patient with acute myeloid leukaemia is seen in clinic with a new onset disseminated rash consisting of juicy red-purple plaques. An incisional biopsy shows a dense neutrophilic infiltrate throughout the dermis. What is the likely diagnosis:

A  Sweet's syndrome
B  paraneoplastic prebullous pemphigoid
C  erythema multiforme
D  leukaemic infiltration
E  lichen planus.

**211** Examining a H&E stained skin biopsy of a lesion you see numerous uniform blue coloured cells which have little cytoplasm, dark oval nuclei and resemble the basal cells of the epidermis. What is the most likely diagnosis:

A   dermatofibroma
B   lichenoid keratosis
C   basal cell carcinoma
D   pyogenic granuloma
E   clear cell acanthoma.

**212** A young male patient presents with a rapidly growing nodule on his thigh. You excise the nodule with narrow margins for a histological diagnosis. Two weeks later you discuss the lesion with the pathologist who comments that the lesion looks highly malignant and is composed of spindle shaped cells, they are awaiting further stains. Which diagnosis is the least likely:

A   sarcoma
B   melanoma
C   squamous cell carcinoma
D   Kaposi's sarcoma
E   Merkel cell carcinoma.

**213** When interpreting a skin biopsy if nuclei are retained in the stratum corneum this is referred to as:

A   parakeratosis
B   papillomatosis
C   orthokeratosis
D   hypergranulosis
E   pseudoepitheliomatous hyperplasia.

**214** You receive a call for advice from a general practitioner who has biopsied a rash on a patient's leg. The biopsy has been reported by a general pathologist who has commented on extensive degenerative collagen. What is the most likely diagnosis:

A   lupus profundus
B   granuloma annulare

C morphea
D lichen sclerosus
E discoid lupus.

**215** A 12-year-old boy presents with a widespread rash shortly after suffering a sore throat. On examination he has numerous small deep red plaques with overlying silvery scale. You suspect a diagnosis of guttate psoriasis. If you were to biopsy the rash which of the following features would you not expect to see:

A increased number and size of capillaries
B epidermal neutrophils
C parakeratosis
D acantholysis
E acanthosis with elongated bulbous rete ridges

**216** You review the biopsy of a rash recently taken from a middle-aged patient. The histopathological features include apoptosis of individual keratinocytes, spongiosis and a lymphocytic vacuolar interface dermatitis. The most likely diagnosis is:

A erythema multiforme
B atopic eczema
C lichen planus
D discoid lupus
E erythema nodosum.

**217** A skin biopsy is taken from a patient with suspected macular amyloidosis. On H&E stained sections there is an amorphous, eosinophilic fissured mass. Congo red staining is likely to reveal:

A a green colour on light microscopy and orange-red birefringence under polarised light
B no staining on light microscopy and green birefringence under polarised light
C an orange-red colour on light microscopy and polarised light
D an orange-red colour on light microscopy and green birefringence under polarised light
E no staining.

**218** A four-year-old girl is brought into A&E with a non-blanching purpuric rash, pyrexia and lethargy. She is diagnosed with suspected meningococcal septicaemia and admitted. The paediatric team request a skin biopsy as initial blood cultures are sterile. If meningococci are present on the skin biopsy what colour would they stain with gram stain:

A   yellow
B   black
C   red
D   blue
E   they will not stain.

**219** A 66-year-old man presents to the chest physicians with an enlarged supraclavicular lymph node. The lymph node is excised and pathologically shows a malignant tumour which stains strongly with the S100 stain. The patient is referred to dermatology with a presumed diagnosis of metastatic malignant melanoma. Apart from malignant melanoma which of the following differential diagnosis should you consider:

A   leiomyosarcoma
B   gastric adenocarcinoma
C   small cell cancer of the lung
D   Merkel cell carcinoma
E   Cholangiocarcinoma.

**220** An 80-year-old lady presents with a growing, bleeding mass on her scalp. Ten years previously she had received radiotherapy to this area for a basal cell carcinoma. Biopsy shows a malignant tumour that stains positively for vimentin, CD31 and CD34. The most likely diagnosis is:

A   squamous cell carcinoma
B   metastatatic breast carcinoma
C   basal cell carcinoma
D   epithelioma cuniculatum
E   angiosarcoma.

**221** A 25-year-old patient of Caribbean descent presents with patchy hair loss. On examination you note a scarring alopecia with some hyperkeratosis. You suspect discoid lupus and perform an incisional biopsy through the edge of a lesion. Which part of the biopsy would you send for direct immune-fluorescence (IMF) and in what medium:

A   lesional skin sent in formaldehyde
B   lesional skin sent in sterile water
C   lesional skin sent in Michel's media
D   peri-lesional skin sent in sterile water
E   peri-lesional skin sent in Michel's media.

**222** You are reviewing a biopsy of a squamous cell carcinoma and discussing the atypical cells with the pathologist. What feature would you not expect to see:

A   hypochromatism
B   hyperchromatism
C   prominent nucleoli
D   abnormal mitoses
E   pleomorphism.

## ANSWERS

### 203 D. Drug exanthem

The histopathology report is of a superficial perivascular dermatitis. Lymphocytes migrate from the superficial blood vessels into the dermis causing this common, non-specific pattern. The pattern is seen in nearly all inflammatory skin diseases.

Causes of a superficial perivascular dermatitis:
- non-specific erythemas
- drug reactions
- viral eruptions
- chronic eczema.

Another common pattern is a superficial and deep perivascular dermatitis, where the inflammation continues down into the deep dermis. This pattern is also non-specific and can be seen in nearly any inflammatory skin disease.

Causes of a superficial and deep perivascular dermatitis:
- causes of a superficial perivascular dermatitis (*see* above)
- papular urticaria (insect bites)
- lupus.

In this question a drug exanthem is the most likely cause of the superficial perivascular dermatitis. Leukaemia cutis often shows a diffuse or nodular pattern with a dense infiltrate of leukaemic cells. A similar dense pattern of infiltrating cells is seen in the tumour stage of mycosis fungoides (cutaneous T-cell lymphoma). Erythema nodosum is characterised by a septal panniculitis, inflammation within the subcutaneous fatty tissues. In Sweet's syndrome a dense neutrophilic infiltrate is seen spreading down from the superficial dermis.

### 204 A. Granuloma annulare

In this question the pathologist is describing a lichenoid interface dermatitis, a dense band of inflammatory cells infiltrating the superficial dermis next to the dermal-epidermal junction (DEJ). This infiltrate can damage the DEJ making it indistinct and creating vacuolar spaces and eosinophilic (pink) blobs – colloid bodies.

Causes of a lichenoid interface dermatitis:
- lichen planus
- lichenoid drug reactions
- lichenoid keratosis

- lupus
- tumour related – Bowen's, melanoma-in-situ.

A vacuolar interface dermatitis is a similar pattern but with a less impressive inflammatory infiltrate.

Causes of a vacuolar interface dermatitis:
- dermatomyositis
- lichen sclerosus
- lupus
- erythema multiforme.

Granuloma annulare is the correct answer as it does not show an interface dermatitis pattern. It is characterised by infiltrating or palisading granulomas (histiocytes/macrophages) and focal degeneration of collagen (necrobiosis).

### 205 E. Mastocytosis

In this case a young child is presenting with an extensive rash and a biopsy showing a diffuse dense infiltrate of monomorphous cells. The pathological patterns of nodular and diffuse dermatitis are often considered together.

Causes of a diffuse/nodular dermatitis:
- granulomatous disorders (*see* question 208)
- infiltration by leukaemia or lymphoma cells
- infections including cellulitis
- mastocytosis
- Sweet's syndrome.

In this question mastocytosis is the most likely answer. In this case the patient has a history of wheeze which may be a systemic feature of mastocytosis and can be incorrectly diagnosed as asthma. Pathologically there is a dense dermal infiltration of monomorphous mast cells with oval nuclei, abundant cytoplasm and basophilic granules. Mast cells stain with toluidine blue, giemsa and chloroacetate esterase.

Nummular eczema shows typical pathological features of spongiosis, intraepidermal oedema and a lymphocytic infiltrate. The features of lupus are variable and include keratinocyte damage, follicular plugging, hyperkeratosis and a lymphohistiocytic infiltrate which may have an interface, periadnexal or diffuse/nodular pattern. Lichen planus would show a lichenoid interface dermatitis pattern. Erythema multiforme would show keratinocyte apoptosis, spongiosis and a vacuolar interface dermatitis.

## 206 C. Staphylococcal scalded skin syndrome

In this question the intentionally vague history points towards a vesiculobullous disorder. The pathology confirms this showing a subcorneal split, a very high split in the epidermis just below the corneocyte layer. There are only a few causes of such superficial bullae.

Causes of subcorneal vesiculobullae:
- staphylococcal infection – bullous impetigo, staphylococcal scalded skin syndrome
- pemphigus foliaceus and erythematosus
- friction blisters.

Superficial blisters may also occur due to a split within the epidermis itself – the intraepidermal vesiculobullous disorders.

Causes of intraepidermal vesiculobullae:
- spongiotic – eczemas
- degenerative – herpes virus infections
- acantholytic disorders (*see* below)
- friction blisters.

Acantholysis is a descriptive term for loss of cohesion between keratinocytes, it is characteristic for a small number of dermatoses:

Acantholytic dermatoses:
- pemphigus vulgaris
- Grover's disease
- Hailey-Hailey disease
- Darier disease.

Porphyria cutanea tarda, bullous pemphigoid and bullous lupus show a deep split at the dermal-epidermal junction. Pemphigus vulgaris is an acantholytic disorder with an intraepidermal split. Staphylococcal scalded skin syndrome is the only disorder in the question with a superficial subcorneal split and is the most likely answer.

## 207 B. Bullous erythema multiforme

In this scenario a patient has developed a subepidermal vesiculobullous disorder soon after being treated with antibiotics for a tonsilar infection. There are a number of causes of subepidermal vesiculobullous disorders and they can be classified according to the locally dominant inflammatory cell type.

**Table 11.1** Disorders that cause subepidermal vesiculobullae

| Inflammatory infiltrate | Disorders associated with |
|---|---|
| Few inflammatory cells | Bullous pemphigoid, porphyrias, diabetic bullae, epidermolysis bullosa acquisita |
| Eosinophilic infiltrate | Bullous pemphigoid |
| Lymphocytic infiltrate | Bullous erythema multiforme, bullous drug eruptions |
| Neutrophilic infiltrate | Linear IgA disease, dermatitis herpetiformis, bullous lupus erythematosus |

In the question the subepidermal split is too deep for either type of pemphigus or staphylococcal scalded skin syndrome and the lymphocytic infiltrate favours erythema multiforme over bullous pemphigoid. Bullous erythema multiforme is a rare manifestation of erythema multiforme but the causes remain the same, in this case either infection (the quinsy) or the antibiotics.

### 208 E. Dermatomyositis
An inflammatory infiltrate composed primarily of histiocytes (macrophages) is termed granulomatous. This pattern of inflammation is specific to a small number of conditions.
    Causes of a granulomatous dermatitis:
- ruptured cysts or follicles
- foreign body granulomas
- xanthogranulomas and xanthomas
- mycobaterial and deep fungal infections
- granuloma annulare
- sarcoidosis.

In this question all the potential answers are granulomatous disorders with the exception of dermatomyositis which is characterised by an interface dermatitis and mucin deposition.

### 209 D. Pustular rash
A collection of neutrophils in the epidermis often presents as a subcorneal pustule. This may either be sterile or infected depending on the pathology of the underlying disorder.
    Causes of neutrophils in the epidermis:
- impetigo, bacterial and mycobacterial infections

227

- fungal and candidal infections
- acne vulgaris
- folliculitis
- psoriasis
- pustular dermatoses of infancy.

## 210 A. Sweet's syndrome

A dermal neutrophilic infiltrate is seen in Sweet's syndrome, a rare neutrophilic dermatoses that is strongly associated with myeloid line haematological malignancies.

Causes of a dermal neutrophilic infiltrate:
- infectious diseases
- some of the subepidermal blistering disorders
- ruptured cysts or follicles
- vasculitis
- the neutrophilic dermatoses.

The neutrophilic dermatoses are a group of disorders characterised by a neutrophilic infiltrate without secondary infection.

The neutrophilic dermatoses:
- pyoderma gangrenosum
- Sweet's syndrome
- Behçet's disease
- inflammatory bowel disease related.

Of the possible answers only Sweet's syndrome is characterised by a significant neutrophilic infiltrate. In prebullous pemphigoid there is often a non-specific infiltrate of lymphocytes and eosinophils, erythema multiforme and lichen planus have a lymphocytic infiltrate and leukaemia cutis is characterised by an infiltration of leukaemic cells.

## 211 C. Basal cell carcinoma

The description is of basaloid cells. These cells resemble the cells found in the basal layer of the epidermis. They have a dark, oval nucleus, little cytoplasm and are basophilic. Basophilic cells are dark blue with H&E staining.

Lesions with a basaloid cell type:
- basal cell carcinoma
- adnexal tumours
- seborrhoeic keratosis.

There are many patterns of basal cell carcinoma all consisting of basaloid cells. Other common features are clefting – a splitting of the sample at the edges of the tumour, and palisading – where the cells line up like the basal layer of the epidermis.

Dermatofibromas are dermal proliferations consisting of spindle shaped fibroblasts and myofibroblasts. Lichenoid keratosis have a characteristic lichenoid interface dermatitis pattern. Pyogenic granulomas consist of lobules of small capillaries in a fibromyxoid matrix. Clear cell acanthomas have a psoriasiform histology with clear/pale keratinocytes. In this question the only lesion that contains basaloid cells is a basal cell carcinoma.

## 212 E. Merkel cell carcinoma
The history is of a rapidly growing malignancy presenting with spindle shaped cells. There are a number of benign and malignant dermatological lesions that consists of spindle shaped cells.

Lesions that may consist of spindle cells:
- benign fibrous proliferations e.g. dermatofibroma
- squamous cell carcinoma
- malignant melanoma
- smooth muscle neoplasms and sarcomas
- neural tumours
- vascular proliferations including Kaposi's sarcoma.

All of the potential answers for this question could fit the history of a rapidly growing malignant nodule. In addition sarcoma, melanoma, squamous cell carcinoma and Kaposi's sarcoma can all occur as spindle cell proliferations. Whereas Merkel cell carcinoma consists of uniform small round/oval cells with ovoid nuclei.

## 213 A. Parakeratosis
In normal epithelium keratinocytes lose their nucleus as they ascend higher in the epidermis, this is called orthokeratosis. If the nucleus is retained and appears in the corneocyte layer it is called parakeratosis. Parakeratosis is a common finding especially in scaly skin disorders.

Dermatoses with parakeratosis:
- psoriasis and pityriasis rubra pilaris (PRP)
- eczema
- actinic keratosis and Bowen's disease
- verruca vulgaris
- tinea.

Pseudoepitheliomatous hyperplasia is an extreme form of epidermal hyperplasia with a grossly thickened epidermis that can be difficult to distinguish from carcinoma. Hypergranulosis refers to thickening of the granular layer and often accompanies hyperkeratosis, it is a non-specific finding that may occur in any hyperkeratotic disorder or lesion. Papillomatosis refers to an irregular undulation of the whole epidermis.

### 214 B. Granuloma annulare
Necrobiosis is characterised by degenerative collagen on histopathology, there are only a few conditions with this feature.

Dermatoses exhibiting necrobiosis:
- necrobiosis lipodica diabeticorum
- granuloma annulare
- rheumatoid nodules.

In this question granuloma annulare is the only disorder that shows necrobiosis. Discoid lupus is characterised by hyperkeratosis, follicular plugging and a lymphocytic infiltrate. Lupus profundus is a predominantly lobular panniculitis. Lichen sclerosus shows a thinned epidermis with a vacuolar interface dermatitis. The pathology of morphea is variable depending on the stage of the disease and where the biopsy is taken from, often little or no changes are seen.

### 215 D. Acantholysis
The features of psoriasis and psoriasiform dermatoses are well recognised. Acantholysis is not a feature of psoriasis, it is a descriptive term for loss of cohesion between keratinocytes and is seen in a small number of disorders as *see* question 206.

Key pathological features of psoriasis:
- increased number and size of capillaries
- migration of neutrophils into the epidermis
- parakeratosis and hypogranulosis
- acanthosis with elongated bulbous rete ridges
- marked mixed perivascular infiltrate.

Hypogranulosis is a decreased thickness of the granular layer of the epidermis, it is strongly associated with parakeratosis *see* question 213. Acanthosis is a thickened spinous layer of the epidermis and usually occurs alongside hyperkeratosis, a thickened stratum corneum layer.

## 216 A. Erythema multiforme

In this question the pathological description is typical of established erythema multiforme.

**Table 11.2** Dermatopathology of common conditions

| Disorder | Histopathological features |
|---|---|
| Eczema | • Spongiosis<br>• Intraepidermal oedema +/− vesicles<br>• Lymphocytic infiltrate<br>• May have parakeratosis and epithelial hyperplasia |
| Discoid lupus | • Keratinocyte damage<br>• Hyperkeratosis<br>• Pronounced lympho-histiocytic infiltrate which may be dermal, interface, perivascular or periadnexal<br>• Follicular plugging |
| Erythema nodosum | • Septal panniculitis |
| Psoriasis | • Increased number and size of capillaries<br>• Oedema at top of papillae<br>• Marked mixed perivascular infiltrate<br>• Epidermal neutrophils +/− microabscesses<br>• Acanthosis, agranulocytosis, parakeratosis and spongiosis |
| Lichen planus | • Lichenoid interface dermatitis with colloid bodies<br>• Lymphocytic infiltrate<br>• Pigmentary incontinence |
| Erythema multiforme | • Apoptosis individual keratinocytes<br>• Spongiosis<br>• Vacuolar degeneration<br>• Lymphocytic infiltrate |

## 217 D. An orange-red colour on light microscopy and green birefringence under polarised light

Amyloid is an amorphous material that can deposit in the skin leading to a variety of clinical appearances. In answer to the question Congo red stains amyloid an orange-red colour and under polarised light green birefringence is seen. There are a number of other stains used for amyloid including crystal violet, methyl violet, PAS and Sirius red.

**Table 11.3** Stains used for deposits and connective tissues

| Stain | Staining |
|---|---|
| Haematoxylin and eosin (H&E) | Nuclei stain blue, cytoplasm stains pink |
| Verhoeff-van Gieson | Elastic tissue stains black, collagen stains red, muscle and nerves stain yellow |
| Congo red | Amyloid stains orange-red and under polarised light green birefringence is seen |
| PAS | Glycogen, neutral polysaccharides, fibrin, hyaline, fungi and basement membranes are stained red |
| Toluidine blue | Mast cell granules and acid mucopolysaccharides stain purple |
| Perl's, Turnbull, and Prussian blue | All stain iron and haemosiderin blue |

## 218 C. Red

Neisseria meningitides is a gram negative diplococcus. Gram positive bacteria stain blue and gram negative bacteria stain pink-red.

**Table 11.4** Stains used for infectious organisms

| Stain | Staining |
|---|---|
| Gram stain | Gram positive bacteria stain blue, gram negative bacteria stain pink-red |
| Ziehl-Neelsen, Fite and Kinyoun's | Acid fast bacilli stain red |
| PAS | Fungal walls are stained red |
| Giemsa | Histoplasma, rickettsia, leishmania and some other bacteria stain purple-blue |

## 219 A. Leiomyosarcoma

S100 stains a calcium binding protein that is expressed in melanocytes and melanocytic tumours. However it is not specific for melanocytes, it also stains glial and Schwann cell tumours, granular cell tumours, eccrine coil neoplasms, Langerhans cells, chondrocytes, smooth and skeletal muscle and their tumours, sarcomas and occasionally breast adenocarcinoma.

Stains for malignant melanoma:
- S100 – sensitive but not specific

- HMB45 – highly specific but poorly sensitive
- Melan-A/MART-1 – specific but poorly sensitive.

In this question leiomyosarcoma is a rare sarcoma of smooth muscle lineage that often stains positive with S100.

## 220 E. Angiosarcoma

In this question the history of a bleeding malignant lesion occurring in a site of previous radiotherapy is suspicious for angiosarcoma. Squamous cell carcinoma may also occur in sites of previous radiotherapy and recurrent basal cell carcinoma remains a possibility, as does a new primary or metastatic lesion. Although vimentin is a non-specific marker, CD31 and CD34 are both highly sensitive markers of vascular tumours such an angiosarcoma.

**Table 11.5** Staining of cancers

| Stain | Staining |
| --- | --- |
| Vimentin | A non-specific stain which stains most tissues of mesenchymal origin – fibroblasts, muscle, endothelial, lymphocytes, histiocytes, melanocytes, Schwann cells. It is useful to exclude tumours which it does not stain – adenocarcinomas and epithelial tumours |
| S100 | Stains melanocytic and neural tumours. *See* question 219 |
| Smooth muscle actin | A marker for myogenic soft tissue tumours and smooth muscle differentiation, it is positive in sarcomas and fibrohistiocytic tumours |
| CD31 | A sensitive marker for vascular tumours |
| CD34 | A less sensitive marker for vascular tumours, also positive in dermatofibrosarcoma protuberans (DFSP), leukaemia, lymphoma |
| CD45 | Positive in most leukaemias and lymphomas |
| Desmin | Stains skeletal and smooth muscle tumours |

## 221 E. Peri-lesional skin sent in Michel's media

Immunoglobulin deposits in the skin are a valuable source of diagnostic information. Best results are usually obtained from peri-lesional skin that has been transported in Michel's media, phosphate-buffered normal saline or Zeuss media. When received, samples are frozen and stained with fluorecein isothiocynate labelled antibodies to IgG, IgM, IgA, C3 and fibrin.

Direct immune-fluorescence (IMF) is useful in:
• immunobullous disorders
• lupus
• vasculitis.

## 222 A. Hypochromatism

Atypical cells are often found in malignancies but may also be found in premalignant and benign lesions. The pathologist needs to interpret atypical cells in the context of their overall architecture, cell type and clinical situation when interpreting if a lesion is malignant.

Features of atypical cells include:
• hyperchromatism – degenerative nuclei with increased pigmentation
• pleomorphism – variability in the size and shape of cells
• prominent nucleoli
• increased nuclear to cytoplasmic ratio
• abnormal mitoses.

In this question hypochromatism is not a commonly seen feature of malignant cells, hyperchromatism is.

# Index

235